W9-AAV-567

MAKING UP

MAKING UP
by REX

Beauty for Every Age, Every Woman

Written by Diana Lewis Jewell
Illustrations by Rex

CLARKSON POTTER/PUBLISHERS

NEW YORK

Text copyright © 1986 by Rex Hilverdink and Diana Lewis Jewell
Illustrations copyright © 1986 by Rex Hilverdink

All rights reserved. No part of this book may be reproduced
or transmitted in any form or by any means, electronic or
mechanical, including photocopying, recording, or by any
information storage and retrieval system, without permission
in writing from the publisher.

Published by Clarkson N. Potter, Inc., 201 East 50th Street,
New York, New York 10022.
Member of the Crown Publishing Group.
CLARKSON N. POTTER, POTTER, and logo are trademarks of
Clarkson N. Potter, Inc.

Manufactured in Hong Kong
Designed by Rochell Udell and Rise Daniels

Library of Congress Cataloging-in-Publication Data
Rex.
    Making up.
1. Beauty, Personal.   2. Cosmetics.
3. Face—Care and hygiene.   I. Jewell,
Diana Lewis.   II. Title.
RA778.R447   1986   646.7'26   85-12441
ISBN 0-517-55754-1
        0-517-56955-8 (pbk.)

10 9 8 7 6 5 4

To Helene Jacobs and Ella May Lewis, forever beautiful.

CONTENTS

Preface 1

Introduction—Rex's Rules 2

1.
A BEAUTY ENVIRONMENT 7
Indispensable Makeup Tools 9

The Minimum Makeup to Own 12

Shopping for Your Makeup 14

Makeup Formulations 16

2.
CARING FOR YOUR SKIN 19
Your Skin Type 20

To Tone or Not to Tone? 24

Moisturizing: A Must 24

Taking Makeup Off 25

Special Care: Skin Care for Changing Seasons 27

3.
HARMONY OF COLOR 29
Your Natural Colors 30

Working with Your Natural Colors 32

Working Around Your Natural Colors 35

Gray Face Remedies 37

4.
FORM OF FACE 39

The Basic Face Shapes 40
Understanding Dark and Light 43
Base Shading 46
The Face Finder 48
Correcting Techniques: Eyebrows 56
Correcting Techniques: Nose 59
Correcting Techniques: Undereye Bags 61
Correcting Techniques: Eyes 62
Correcting Techniques: Forehead and Jawline 66
Correcting Techniques: Lips 67
Step by Step to a Perfect Makeup 70

5.
CHARACTER OF FACE 75

Fashion and Makeup 76
The Three Faces of Fashion 78
A Round-the-Clock Makeup Strategy 86
Beauty for Every Age 90
Tips to Look 10 Years Better 105
Makeup for Black Women 107
Makeup for Asian Women 109
Makeup for Women with White Hair 110
Makeup for Women Who Wear Eyeglasses 112
Fantasy Makeup 114
Planet Faces 118

Acknowledgments 124

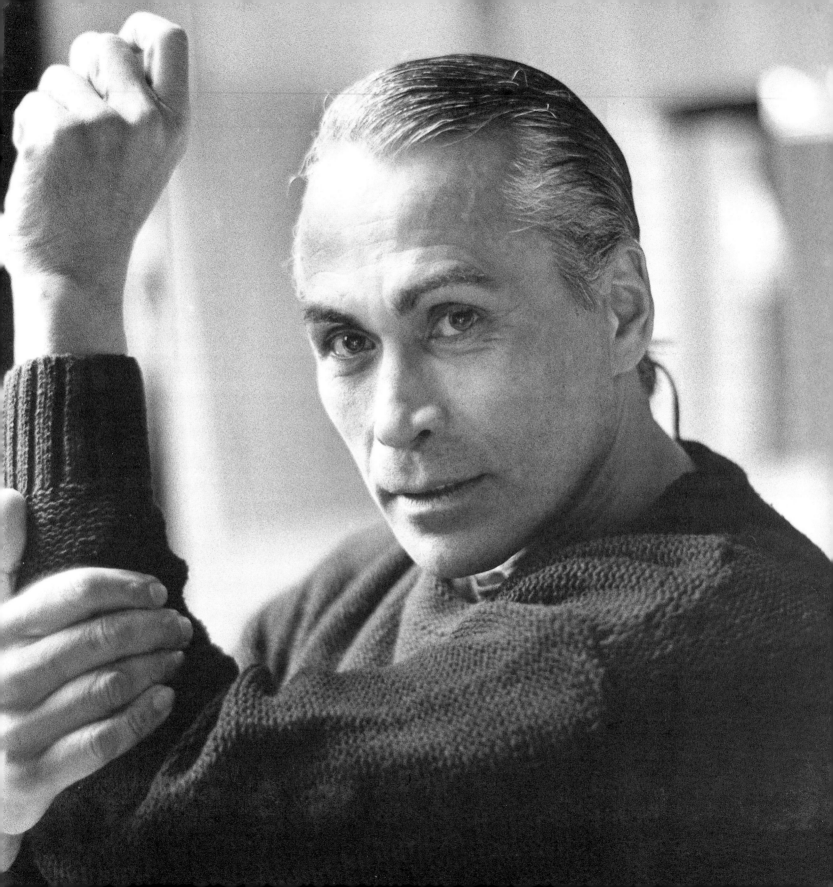

PREFACE

For me, makeup is something I fell into by the sheerest accident. My first love was dance, and I spent several years touring Europe with ballet and modern dance troupes. Even then, however, I was fascinated by the play of dark and light, lines and colors, and I spent many of my spare hours trying to recapture the magic of the faces I saw on stage in sketches.

When, in 1970, my dancing career was cut short by an injury, I wondered if I couldn't make professional use of my drawing ability. On a whim, I brought a handful of sketches to the Elizabeth Arden salon in Paris, where I was then living. The salon was at that time being run by Miss Arden's sister, the Vicomtesse de Maublanc. What she said to me changed my life forever. After looking through all of my sketches, she announced decisively, "If you can do these, you can design great makeup." It was then that I began a career that has given me the greatest pleasure and success.

After establishing myself as a makeup artist with the Arden salon in Paris and throughout France, I joined an international cosmetics company as *chef maquilleur*. That is when an editor at French *Vogue* convinced me to go out on my own as a free-lance makeup artist for fashion and beauty shootings. That very year I did my first *Vogue* cover and within two years I was working on both sides of the Atlantic.

Doing so many faces in a short period of time, I soon learned quite a bit about making a woman beautiful—and, more important—about making her *feel* beautiful. All of us, no matter how plain we may consider ourselves, have at least one feature we are secretly proud of. This is the feature I focus on when I am creating a makeup; playing up a finely sculpted lip, or deep, sultry eyes. Even if the application is more intense than the woman is used to, I know she'll respond positively. And getting a woman to change the way she does her makeup, to consider colors and techniques she's never dared to try before is what makes my job exciting. I think makeup is like a party—it should make explosions, make fun, and most of all, be a vivid, vibrant expression of the woman inside.

Rex Hilverdink
New York, New York 1986

INTRODUCTION— REX'S RULES

Have you ever imagined what it would be like to have your face completely, professionally "done" by a famous makeup artist? Well, allow me to do you. I'll introduce you to all the beautiful tricks I've used on hundreds of top cover models—and I'll let you in on them step by step. I'll explain each technique as if it were a private beauty lesson. And I'll suggest new things to try that you may have thought could never work for you. The best part is, it's going to be easier than you ever imagined!

It's not such a complicated task to develop your maximum beauty potential. There really are no closely guarded secrets, no tricks the "pros" keep only to themselves. There are no miracle formulas hidden behind the doors of the world's most exclusive salons. There is no mystery. There are simply basic techniques. And they *can* be learned.

If you haven't been able to teach yourself the steps to a beautiful makeup before now, maybe you've had the wrong teacher. Picking up bits of information here and there is no way to go about it. It's best to follow a single, simple system, with unified advice. Mixing techniques will give you mixed results—at best.

Sometimes the clock gets more blame for a makeup disaster than the cosmetics do. The most popular rationale I hear when a woman isn't satisfied with the way she looks is, "I didn't have time this morning." Translation: She's not to blame; her schedule is. Don't you believe it. No matter how tight your schedule is, you can still do the right things for your face. But whether it takes five minutes or a luxuriant half-hour, the entire process will produce the results you want only if you know what you're doing. The myth that it takes more time to do a "professional" job is just that—a myth. You can waste twenty minutes with the wrong attempts, just as easily as you can fill them with the right techniques. It's the same twenty minutes—but what a difference!

It's important to be able to live up to your beauty potential—for your own self-esteem and for reasons that go beyond vanity. Knowing what you're doing may literally save your face. Careless application or selection of the wrong beauty products may do damage to your skin. If you are going to put makeup on and take makeup off almost every day of your adult life, you owe it to yourself to learn how to do it right.

What do you want from your mirror? Just what are your expectations when you put on makeup? Honesty? Fantasy? A blending of both? Someone you don't even recognize? Think about it for a moment. These questions are not as frivolous as you may think. Are you simply preparing "a face to meet the faces that you meet"? Are you hiding anything? Are you going for glamour? Are you underlining your personality? Are you trying to project a different personality? Do you strive to appear fashionable? Changeable? Unpredictable? Or do you try never to change? In the midst of passing fads, do you like your look to remain steadfast, loyal, and true? Does age affect your strategy—a desire to look younger or older? Do you wear makeup only for special occasions? Or only on bad days?

There are probably as many reasons, deep down, for women wearing makeup as there are women wearing makeup. Analyzing your motivation will give you a clue to why you apply your makeup the way you do. In general, women who wish to change (age, personality, general facial characteristics) overdo the amount of makeup they use and the way they apply it. And women who are satisfied with the status quo—or women who are afraid of makeup or of change—often underemphasize their best features.

What's needed is a *balance* between what is and what could be. The blending of your own features with the image you wish to project requires patient retouching. A sudden shock of color isn't going to do it. Nor is the instant creation of a whole new face. If the structure doesn't change, you end up merely applying artificialities—and they will be found out.

The synthesis you are after, the balance of truth and illusion, requires an honest appraisal, a bit of research, and a willingness to experiment. To be free to create, you need to open yourself up to new possibilities without denying the realities. They are what make you *you*.

You've got to go with what you've got, and make the most of it. Nothing more, nothing less will do.

Self-knowledge is the first crucial step in creating an image close to your personal ideal. Once you have established an equilibrium between the "real" you deep inside and the image you want others to see, you can begin to explore the possibilities of makeup. You can make decisions on the basis of intelligence, not wishful thinking. You can discover the power of your own potential, instead of relying on impersonal beauty formulas. You can communicate the variability of your own personality.

When you apply makeup, you become an artist. No masterpiece is ever created unless the artist understands the medium he or she is working with. An artist knows which materials accept color and how readily, which colors create shadows, which ones bring something out of hiding. An artist knows how to prime the canvas for even application, how to create a wash of colors to suggest transparency, how to fix color for maximum adherence.

Every morning, when you first touch your face, you are in a sense becoming an artist. Your face is your canvas, your skin is its texture, your makeup is your medium. And you need to understand how they all work together: how skin affects makeup, how color affects shape, how shape affects placement, how character affects color selection. Everything is interrelated, and if you are unsure about even one of these elements, you may end up missing your image by a mile—even if you've only gone wrong by a shade! Something as simple as a lipstick that's too aggressively bright may throw your whole appearance out of kilter. Unless you know the principles behind creating a successful makeup, it's easy to make a mistake without knowing why.

The real secret to choosing the correct makeup is to understand the underlying principles of *color, form,* and *character.* Once you know these, you are free to create, not to experiment blindly. There's a big difference. I'll tell you how to make these principles work for you later in the book, but right now it is enough to be aware of these three important factors.

Harmony of Color

Nothing adds excitement to the face more than color. It creates a mood, expresses a definite personality. But it must be part of the whole picture. You want the colors you choose for your makeup to be compatible with your own personal coloring, as well as appropriate for the shades you like to wear. The idea is to create a total harmony of color. When everything is "in sync," the end result is that much more attractive.

Form of Face

The form of your face is, irrevocably, deter-

REX'S REALISTIC BEAUTY RULES

Makeup can be—and should be—many things. But the one thing it should never be is obvious. If someone admires your makeup, it is not a compliment. If someone admires your beauty, you've succeeded. The guidelines below will help you cross the line from a beautiful makeup to a beautiful face.

Don't Hide Behind Your Makeup
Makeup is not a mask. It is meant to enhance your beauty, not overwhelm it.

Be Original
Unique features should not always be considered imperfections. Instead of "correcting" distinctive characteristics through shading, make them part of your beauty.

Follow Through
Don't think you can make up only one part

of your face. If you're going to do your eyes, you have to do the rest; otherwise, you will be placing too much emphasis on a single part of your face.

Blend Everything
Never just apply makeup and leave it there. Always blend, blot, or brush everything.

Don't Be a One-Color Woman
Avoid being typecast by your colors. Learn how to work within different harmony-of-color schemes.

Keep It Subtle
Guard against overdoing makeup. Extremes of color and application can take over your face. Less is *always* more.

Wear the Right Face at the Right Time
Plan an appropriate makeup for every activity. One wear-with-everything face really goes with nothing.

mined by the bones you were born with. Short of major surgical reconstruction, nothing is going to alter this aspect of your appearance. You can change your nose, you can tuck up your chin, you can unpuff your eyes, but the basic shape of your face just isn't going to change. To plan the most attractive makeup for you, it is essential that you learn how to work within the confines of your basic facial structure—both to emphasize your assets and to compensate for any shortcomings.

Character of Face

It is human nature to look for personality clues in the structure of a face. Typecasting though it may be, we see a certain personality in the set of a jaw, the arch of an eyebrow, the tilt of a nose. Determining the character of your own face will influence your makeup *selection* as much as the form of your face influences makeup *placement.* For instance, you would not select overly bright colors for an essentially serious visage. You wouldn't go overly dramatic with a jovial, round face. You don't need to overpower a very strong face. And you shouldn't let the sweetness suggested by an oval face get lost with somber shades.

With makeup, you can express any look you wish to convey: sunny, dramatic, moody, innocent, natural. With skillful application, you can make the subtle changes that will keep you current, update your beauty look. With a bit of imagination, you can create fantasy when you want a little magic. Once you know what you want from makeup at any given moment, the real joy of discovering *all* your faces awaits you.

There is no limit, no one formula. There are times when you'll want to rethink everything, times when you'll accentuate something, times when you'll blend it away. But the power to create the exact effect you want will be in your hands—and in your head. Because beauty is, above all, a matter of intelligence. What beauty products you select, when you choose to use them, and the techniques you employ are all a function of informed investigation and careful editing. In the final analysis, how you choose to let the world see you is an expression from the very heart and soul. It is one of the most personal decisions you will make, yet it is there for all the world to see.

I hope this book will guide you in making that decision. In the chapters ahead you will learn why certain shades or certain makeup techniques work for you—and others don't. You'll find out how to recognize facial structure and how to modify it. You will go through a basic makeup application, step by step, then learn how to personalize it to suit your style, your personality, your age. You'll discover professional secrets for correcting less-than-favorable features. You'll explore the world of color and learn that there's no limit to the shades you can wear—*if* you know how to make them work for you. Finally, you'll find fashionable new makeup ideas to try from subtle seasonal changes to all-out fantasy.

You'll find guidelines for the development of your own personal beauty in every chapter of this book. So do read it through *before* you begin to experiment. Armed with all the professional information I can give you, you may consider things you have never tried before. And you're going to make a beautiful discovery. You!

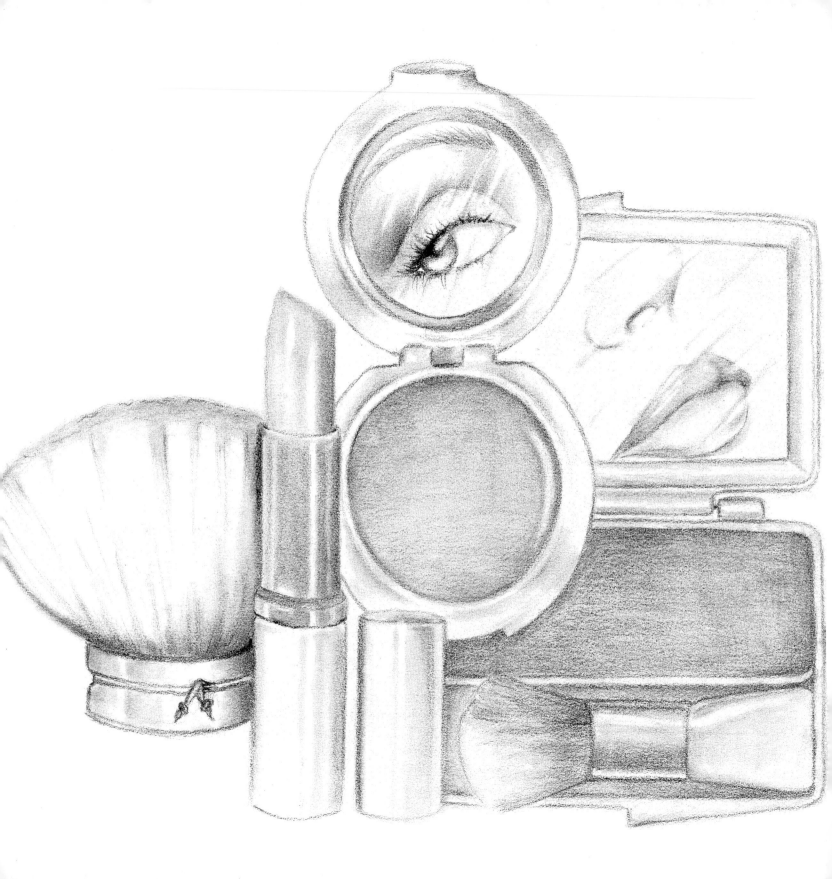

1
A BEAUTY ENVIRONMENT

To create the best makeup, you have to do it
under the best conditions.

Some women put their makeup on in the strangest places: seated in the front of a moving car, riding in a public bus, standing in a line. All the while, they peer into the smallest mirror they can hold in one hand while balancing an applicator in the other. How they can draw a straight line when the car goes around a corner is one mystery; how they can see how one part of the face relates to the other is a different issue altogether.

At one time or another, every woman has "touched up" in a tiny mirror in a public place. But it's hardly the ideal way to start out the day. Not only should you set aside the time to do the job properly; you need to set aside a proper place as well. If you want to look your best in twenty minutes or less, you'll need to have the right tools in the right place for maximum makeup efficiency.

You'll accomplish nothing if you spend the first ten minutes of your time rounding up the makeup supplies you think you'll need. If your favorite mascara is in yesterday's handbag (which one was it?), and your taupe-toned lipstick is in the glove compartment of the car, and your pressed-powder compact is in some pocket or another, you'll never make it in twenty minutes. Even worse, you may settle for whatever you can find! The trick to simplifying the whole process is to create a professional beauty environment. It doesn't have to be elaborate, and you don't need an extra room to do it. But you do need to find an organizable area. Pick one spot and stock it with a permanent collection of supplies.

Where do you usually put on your makeup? In the bathroom? At a dressing table? In a corner of the bedroom? Although you may feel the most comfortable in a certain area, it may not give you the truest reading of how your makeup looks. The mirror may be off. Or there may be no storage capabilities. Or you may have to face fluorescent lighting. None of these situations is ideal. If you want to look your best, you'll need to find the best location. To have an organized, everything-in-one-place makeup area, you'll need an adequate mirror, plenty of shelf and drawer space, and natural lighting. If you can find a spot that has these elements to start with, you're on your way to turning any area into a professional makeup center. Here's what you'll need—and what you'll need to avoid:

HAVE
- a window nearby. You'll need to check or correct your finished look by daylight.

- a mirror surrounded by 25-watt bulbs.

- neutral no-color walls; light gray is best.

- a mirror that angles on the sides.

- ample drawer space, outfitted with organizers.

- specific drawer space for everyday makeup, for special-effects makeup, and for treatment products.

AVOID
- fluorescent light; it takes a lot of the red tones away.

- lights that are directly overhead; they create confusing shadows.

- dark walls, bright walls, busy wallpaper.

- a flush-with-the-wall mirror.

- storage space near pipes or near areas subject to hot or cold temperatures.

- clutter, falling objects, jumbles.

Indispensable Makeup Tools

If you're going to create, you need the right tools to do so—*and* you need to know how to use them. Most women, after all, have purchased a lipstick brush at one time or another. Some have an eyelash curler. Virtually all have tweezers. But most have never learned the most professional ways to use them. So before you even begin to think about makeup, collect all the beauty tools you'll need—and learn exactly what they're for.

Cotton Roll

Use a cotton roll to cut your own cotton balls —you can make them any size, any shape you want. Custom-made balls are much more practical than the uniform-sized, prepackaged balls that shrink to nothing when wet. To make your own, simply cut 2- or 3-inch squares of cotton off the roll, and flip the corners under. The cotton will form a ball under water—and it can be used for absolutely everything. Press the water out until the ball is flat, and use it to apply products to the face. It will blend makeup more evenly than a dry cotton ball and is much more hygienic than reusable applicators. A wet-then-pressed cotton ball won't leave "fuzzies" on the face, and because it absorbs little liquid it makes makeup application much more economical. When pressed lightly to the face, it will set loose powder and dab on just the right amount of liquid blusher. Think of this as your primary beauty tool.

Makeup Sponges

Some women prefer to apply makeup base with a sponge. A sponge can create different textures, different coverage. The wetter it is, the more transparent your makeup will be; the drier, the thicker. Look for a sponge with a texture close to your skin's. Wash sponges with soap and rinse them with water after each use; then let them dry in the open air.

Cotton Swabs

You can make your own swabs with cotton from a cotton roll wrapped around the end of an orange stick, or you can buy the commercially prepared kind. Either way, they are handy tools for keeping your makeup neat. Use them to clean eye corners, to blend, to correct errors. If you smudge your mascara from your lower lashes to the lid beneath, a cotton swab is just the right size to get in there and clean things up. If you make a mistake outlining your mouth, a cotton swab dipped in cleansing cream will whisk it away without smudging the entire line. Always have a few swabs ready and waiting to come to your rescue when you're doing any makeup. I do— and I use them! If "pros" can make mistakes, you can too.

Tissues

There's no mystery to using tissues. Most women wouldn't put on or take off makeup without a box of tissues nearby to cleanse, to remove excess moisture, to blot. But a tissue should never be used as a cleaning rag. Do not scrub or wipe your face with it. Press it against any excess foundation, powder, or cream, then lift off.

Brushes, Brushes, Brushes

The best way to stroke on color of any kind is with a brush. It gives a much softer application and blends away any harsh lines instantly. But all brushes can't do all things. You'll need a variety of sizes and shapes. Make sure the bristles are soft (sable is best; natural is better than synthetic), well anchored (you don't want tiny hairs shedding all over your face), and clean (wash them in soapy lukewarm water once or twice a month and dry quickly, pressing in a towel). And make sure the shape of the brush is scaled to the job. Brushes for applying creams (undereye concealer and lipstick) should be smaller, tighter, and more tapered. Powder brushes (for blush, powder, and eye shadow) can be full, fluffy, and blunt. You'll need a collection of seven to be completely outfitted:

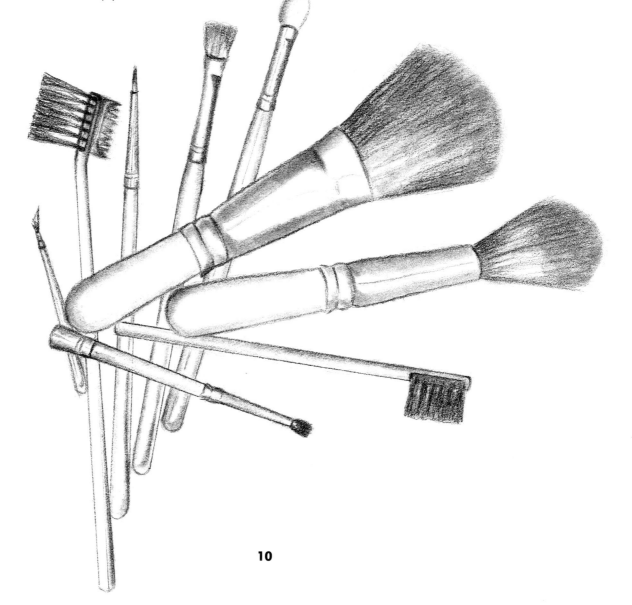

10

BLUSH BRUSH Often of sable hair, indispensable to work with powder blush. The longer the handle, the softer your stroke will be for better blending. (You'll brush harder with a shorter handle.)

MASCARA BRUSH A stiff, thin-bristled brush used to apply cake mascara or separate lashes between coats of mascara. Always rinse completely after each use or mascara will cake between the bristles and make the brush stiff.

LIPSTICK BRUSH A sturdy, short-bristled brush, best when tapered. It can be retractable for easy carrying. Always wipe bristles clean after use.

CONCEALER BRUSH A brush with slanted edges and a replaceable top. This gets right up into the eye corner where the bluish discoloration begins. (Your finger can never reach here without smudging concealer onto the side of your nose!) You can use a lip brush, cutting the edges into a diagonal slant. Wipe the brush clean after every use.

EYEBROW BRUSH/LASH COMB Used wet, dry, or misted with hair spray to tame an unruly browline. The lash comb will "unstick" and separate lashes. This is very important, since clumps make your eyes look dirty and can absolutely ruin even the most beautiful eye makeup! Rinse the lash comb after every use. Clean both the eyebrow brush and the lash comb with soap and water from time to time.

EYELINER BRUSH A very thin brush, often drawn up into a tube. It is used to draw a thin line to modify the shape of the eye.

BLENDING BRUSH A short-bristled brush, usually made of sable or pony hair. It is good for overall blending and for obtaining a softer application of colors.

POWDER BRUSH A big, soft brush used to repowder when makeup is complete. It will eliminate excess powder and leave a transparent finish.

Tweezers

Whether you use straight- or slant-edged tweezers is purely a matter of personal choice. Whichever style you prefer, always make sure your tweezers are able to extract the hair at its base without cutting it. And always clean tweezers after each use with 90-proof alcohol.

Sponge-Tip Applicators

Used for applying and blending eye shadow, sponge-tip applicators give a subtle effect without streaking. Replace applicators often, and use only one per color. Wash them from time to time, pressing the sponge between your fingers to dry. Don't let water remain in the sponge.

Pencil Sharpener

Keep your pencil sharpener clean with 90-proof alcohol, and always sharpen pencils before use to kill the germs. Use a razor blade to create a very flat point for easier application of color to lips and eyes.

The Minimum Makeup to Own

If you love to accumulate all the newest makeup products, all the latest shades, nothing is going to stop you. But you don't need everything on the market to do as much as you want with makeup. You can work wonders with a basic collection of twenty-two products. All the makeup effects in this book (with the exception of fantasy faces) can be achieved by blending and combining the following items.

Bases: 2

Bases give the illusion of perfect skin, unifying the grain and giving it a luminous aspect. To enable your makeup to blend harmoniously with your clothes and coloring, you should be able to take your complexion toward the pink tones and the yellow tones. So you must have both a pink/rose base and a true beige/ivory base.

Buy the best base products you can afford. Remember, this covers most of your face most of the time. Bases of poor quality can dry skin out and imbalance its pH.

Color-Tinted Moisturizers: 2

Tinted moisturizer has the properties of both a moisturizer and a very light base. Depending on the condition of your skin, you may wish to use it instead of a base. It color-corrects the skin's natural tones, unifies the complexion, and gives a very natural appearance when worn alone. But it is not for all women. If you wish to cover any imperfections, you're better off with a base.

If you do choose to wear tinted moisturizer in place of a base, be sure to have one in a pink/rose range and one in a beige/ivory range to make your skin tone compatible with any colors you choose to wear.

Concealers: 2

Concealers can work magic, to cover or to highlight. You'll need two—one a half shade lighter than your base color and one a half shade darker. Use the lighter one to take away shadows and highlight areas that need more "strength" (the bridge of your nose or your chin, for example). Use the darker one to play down unwanted puffiness on either side of a wrinkle or to camouflage blemishes.

Eye Shadows: 3

Unless you love to play with all the shades of the rainbow, you *can* easily get by with only three colors. Choose one in the blue/aqua/mauve/burgundy range; one in the yellow/olive/brown/taupe range; and one good strong neutral, like gray, navy blue, or black.

You can vary the depth of your three basic shades by the way you apply them. Mixing a little water with a powder shadow will give it greater intensity.

Eyeliner Pencils: 3

You can use any type of eye color pencil to line the eye, as long as it is very creamy and very easy to apply. Buy the best products you can find—it's worth the expense to treat the tender skin around the eye gently. A bargain pencil is no bargain. Of course, you may want many colors, but for a minimum makeup, you will need a wardrobe of only three. Choose neutral shades: taupe, gray, and navy if you are fair; brown, black, and burgundy if you are dark.

Eyebrow Pencils: 2

Blending two colors makes your browline more natural. Use either brown and gray or black and gray. Black alone gives too harsh a line; blond is ineffectual; and red is too theatrical. If your eyebrows are very far from the shade you want, have them professionally tinted. Overcompensating for a weak brow with obviously colored pencil will only look harsh.

Mascara: 1

Pick the color closest to that of your natural lashes—and stick with it. Save obvious colors for special occasions.

Lipsticks: 4

You can easily create any lipstick shade you'll need from only three basic colors: pink, red, and a brownish tone. Add a colorless gloss to maximize shine, help blend, and create different looks.

Blushers: 3

You'll need the same basic shades for a wardrobe of blush colors. Invest in a good pink, a red, and a brown-toned contouring blush.

Powder: 1

It's best not to match your powder tints to your base colors. On some days you may want to wear powder alone or powder over a tinted moisturizer. Or you may switch your basic base colors from day to day. The best wear-with-anything powder is transparent, adding absolutely no color.

Compact Powder: 1

Use compact powder for retouching only, not for a powder finish after you have first applied your makeup. You'll need a compact powder to travel with you. Select a shade lighter than your loose powder. Compressed powder always looks a shade darker than it really is.

THE MINIMUM MAKEUP TO TAKE

Any woman who spends more time away from home than she spends at home during the day should have a selection of both makeup and treatment products at her second location. It saves wear and tear on your bag (and on you!) if you don't have to tote a complete makeup collection everywhere you go. You need carry only a blusher, a compact powder, and a lipstick with you if you have the following items tucked into a desk drawer:

1 Moisture stick	2 Eyebrow pencils
2 Bases or tinted moisturizers	1 Mascara
1 Concealer	2 Lipsticks (one pink/mauve, one coral/red)
2 Blushers (one pink, one red)	1 Colorless gloss
3 Eye shadows	1 Brow brush
2 Eyeliner pencils	1 Compact powder

Shopping for Your Makeup

If you're going to go out now and stock up on everything new, you'd better take along your gold credit card! Cosmetics are getting costlier by the minute, and the trend shows no signs of stopping. Your first purchase can be less expensive if you regulate your rate of buying. *NEVER WAIT UNTIL YOU RUN OUT.* When your bottle of beige base is half full, buy a bottle of pinkish base. When your coral blusher is half gone, add a red one to your stock. And so on. The same strategy holds for replacing treatment products.

If you like to sample new shades before you buy, it's best to do your shopping in department stores rather than in drugstores or supermarkets. The stock in department stores is turned over regularly, so the products are usually fresher. And your access to the product is not blocked by blister packaging or locked cases. It's simply easier to test at counters where the main focus is on cosmetics. It's even better when you can find a trained beauty adviser who knows the products backward and forward. If she's gone through the product education classes provided by most major cosmetics companies, she'll be able to assist you with a demonstration of other, compatible products so you can see how the makeup you're trying works best. You may think she's trying to sell you something. I think of it as assistance. Remember, you're not obligated to buy a thing.

You'll need help in trying on new colors or new bases properly. Dabbing a base on the back of your hand tells you nothing. Ask for a moisturizer to rub into your skin, then a dusting of powder to apply on top of your test spot. This will let you see exactly what the base will look like when you wear it.

If you're going to try a new color, ask for a tissue or a sponge with a little cleanser on it to remove the makeup you've already got on. That bright red lipstick you're testing will look much too assertive if you've got a soft pink blusher on or if you're wearing heavy eye makeup. The biggest mistake you can make is to try on new color with old. If you take most of the existing color off your face, and work with a trained adviser, you'll begin to see how the new colors balance one another.

This is not something to do on a lunch hour. You have to plan a time to try on new shades, just as you set aside time to build a new summer or winter wardrobe. If possible, book an appointment so that a beauty adviser can do a complete demonstration on you. You'll learn how shades work with one another. And you'll discover that you may already have many similar shades at home that will balance the few new ones you want.

When you are testing products, especially on your face, make sure everything is clean— brushes, bottles, pencils. Look for alcohol or alcohol wipes next to the brushes. Make sure all pencils are resharpened before testing, and ask for fresh cotton swabs instead of used sponge-tip applicators. Walk away from any salesclerk who wants to touch you with a dirty applicator.

What to Look For

The vast variety of products, formulations, and colors at the counter can seem staggering. Just remember, your first consideration should be the *quality* of the product. Is it fresh? Is it easy to apply? Will it be drying? Here are the things to look for before buying.

Base

Sample base on the back of your hand after moisturizing and powdering over. It should glide on beautifully. If it feels drying, looks chalky, or seems too greasy, you'll know!

Eye Shadow

Eye color should hold true from the case with just one stroke. If you have to rub hard to get the color to come up, you'll have to rub hard on your eyelid too.

Blusher

As with eye shadow, the color should hold up. You shouldn't have to work too hard to obtain a true shade.

Mascara

Remove the wand. If the product clumps around the bristles, don't buy it.

Lipstick

The only way to tell if lipstick is going to be drying is to try it on. But wipe off the entire bullet of the tester tube with a tissue first.

Powder

Roll powder between your fingers. Look for a creamy, light texture. Avoid anything with sparkles; this never looks natural in daylight.

When in Doubt, Pitch It Out

Finding storage places for the makeup and makeup tools you need is no small task if your drawers are cluttered with shades that looked good but weren't. One of the best ways to clear up makeup clutter is to go through your collection—right now—and throw out any makeup you've been "saving." If you don't use shades on a regular basis, you're never going to use them. Also, any products containing oil or cream bases can outlive their "shelf life," spoil, and cause an adverse reaction on your skin. So take the plunge, and throw out:

● any base you haven't used up in six months. The date on the package tells you only how long the product may remain on a retailer's shelf, unopened. Once you begin using it, germs and dust enter with every application.

● any night cream or oil-based moisturizer that has been stored in a warm place.

● any product that smells "off," turns color, or shows signs of oil separation or color separation.

● any mascara that starts drying or becomes "blobby" at the end when you extract the wand. Constantly opening and closing a mascara causes the product to thicken, and then it's finished.

In general, you can worry less about powdery products than about creams and liquids. You can use eye shadows even after you see a slight film on the top. This comes from use, not from spoilage. Simply scratch the film off the top with a pin to get at the fresh color underneath.

Makeup Formulations

There is a difference in the way you approach your face when you are using a cream, a gel, or a powder. Some products can be applied directly to the skin; some never should be. It all depends on their consistency, and on the type of skin you have. A dry or greasy complexion often dictates the type of product you can use. Anything too heavy, too stiff, too unblendable should always go on the hand first, on the face second.

Base

Whichever formulation you choose, never use your fingertips to apply base; it will disappear much sooner than if you use a wet-then-pressed cotton ball or a damp sponge.

LIQUID The most fluid form of coverage. Liquid base gives a fine, supple texture, plus a softer look to the face. It's good for all kinds of skin, and it's the only base to use if your skin is tired.First, place a small circle of base on the back of your hand. Then dip the dampened (and squeezed) cotton ball or sponge into it and apply to your face.

TINTED MOISTURIZER A moisturizing, light base to unify tans and wake up a gray complexion. Tinted moisturizers have greater staying power on normal to dry skin. Add a dusting of transparent powder to make them last longer. Apply only a thin film, using a wet-then-pressed cotton ball.

COMPACT For even greater coverage. This is the least transparent base of all. Be careful not to let it become a mask. Always apply with a damp sponge, and blot with a tissue.

POWDER Less creamy, but more transparent than a compact base. It looks like a powder, but covers like a base. Best for greasy skin or for retouching. Apply with a flat puff or dry cotton square in a rolling, press/release motion.

CREAM Less transparent, more sophisticated coverage. Good for dry skin. Never apply cream with fingertips. Use a damp sponge or a wet-then-pressed cotton ball. Avoid cream base altogether if you have tired skin. Its heavy consistency will emphasize the wrinkles!

Blush

It would be helpful if you could make your face blush naturally to see where the color comes to your cheeks; then you could apply your favorite shade to the spot. But even if you can't, remember that blusher should look as natural as a blush. Put your brush in the blusher, and deposit it *all* exactly where you want to accent, then blend. Do not stroke color on.

CREAM Ideal for dry skin or tanned skin. It slips on easily and has a semi-oily consistency. Never apply it directly to the cheek, or you'll get a shock of color. Work the blush into your hand first, warming it up with your body heat. Apply over moisturizer.

GEL More transparent color, but also a more drying quality. Best for oily skin. A gel can give potent color, and it does not blend easily, so apply it to the hand first. If you put a spot of gel directly on your face, the spot will stay with you all day. Apply over moisturizer.

POWDER Best for moister skins. Never apply a powder blush on dry, unmoisturized skin. You'll get a hot spot of color. Powder is better than cream blush for touch-ups. Use a long-handled brush to keep your hand light.

Eye Shadow

CREAM Not for everybody. Cream shadow should be used only when the eyelid is wrinkle-free and should never be applied to deep-set eyes. If the lid comes in contact with the browbone, body heat will turn the shadow into grease. Also, cream shadow tends to collect in any lines or folds. It creates a dramatic effect, but it's best only on normal-to-dry skin.

POWDER Much more transparent and subtle than other forms of eye color. Powdered shadows are easy to blend and place less stress on the lid. Don't be afraid to coat the applicator with as much color as you can get, so that it goes on in a single, light stroke. Always powder eyelids before applying powder shadow. This gives the color something to cling to. Beware of overly iridescent formulations, which can be aging.

LIQUID Very drying. Unless you have noticeably oily skin, avoid liquid shadow. For easier blending, be sure to apply a moisturizer first.

PENCILS Must be blended to avoid a hard line of color. Never use pencil directly on the eyelids. Stroke color into the palm of your hand to warm it up, then apply it to the lid with a tiny brush. If you are going inside the eye rim with a pencil, always burn the tip of the pencil first to kill germs. Burning also makes the pencil adhere better, so that particles of color are less likely to fall into the eye.

Concealers
Concealers come in creams or solid sticks. Choose the form that is easiest for you to use. Texture is the most important consideration. Whichever form you choose, make sure it has a creamy, blendable consistency.

Mascara
When it comes to selecting which mascara formulation is right for you, you must, of course, consider what you want it to live through. Of equal concern should be the condition of your lash hairs. You don't want to dry them out any more than you would want to dry out the hairs on your head. Cake mascara is best for keeping your lash hairs in good condition. It contains wax, which is much kinder to lashes than the alcohol in some waterproof formulations. The fibers in lash-lengthening mascaras can cause trouble. At the very least, there is little control over where the additional lashes fall. You could get a clump right where you don't want it. If you wish a thicker appearance to your lashes, you'll get better results and have more control if you dust them with powder while one of the mascara layers is still wet.

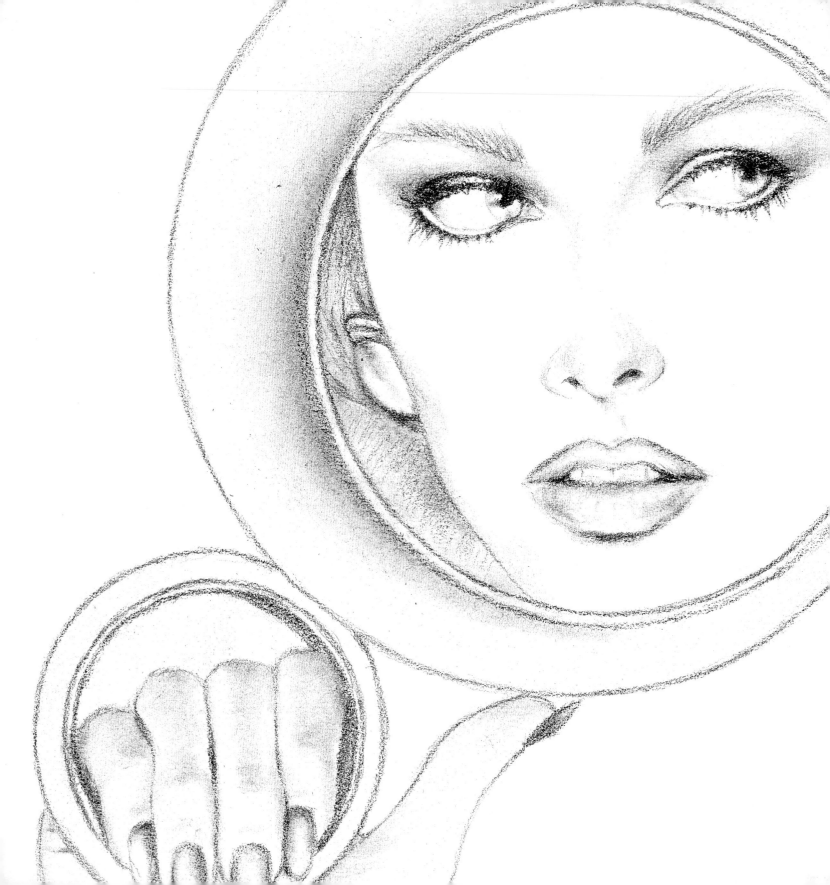

2
CARING FOR YOUR SKIN

Clear skin is the most important beautifier of all—
even if you wear no makeup.

If makeup is your paint, your skin is your canvas. Its texture, its absorbency, its very personality all affect the final, finished picture. There is simply no way you can do a beautiful makeup on badly treated skin.

You must do everything you can to give your skin what it needs. The products you buy, from treatment preparations to makeup and cleansing formulas, should all be determined —first and foremost—by the type of skin you have.

Advertising claims or package promises alone should never influence your choice of which beauty products to buy. *You should think only of doing what's right for your skin.* Every time you choose a cleanser or a cream for any other reason, you are risking disaster. Without a supple, healthy, fresh-looking complexion, your makeup isn't really going to matter. (Of course, there are techniques for correcting "gray face" days and I will explain them later. But as a general rule you shouldn't have to create the illusion of fresh skin.)

Proper cleansing, toning, and moisturizing are the three most important things you will ever do for your skin. It is essential that you develop your own personal ritual of care, based on the discovery of your skin's idiosyncrasies. It may be a trial-and-error process at first, but you should be guided by your honest appraisal of your skin type.

Once you select a treatment product that works for you (a cleanser, for example), try the other products in the same line. It's best if your toner and moisturizer come from the same cosmetics company as your cleanser. That way, you know the formulations all have the same chemical base. When you switch around, selecting a moisturizer from one place and a toner from another, the chemical formulations may not be compatible. And what you perceive as an "allergic" reaction may just be a bad mix.

This doesn't mean that you must stick with one manufacturer for life. In fact, you shouldn't. It does your skin good to switch occasionally. Just make sure, if you are going to an entirely different manufacturer, that you switch all treatment products at the same time. Don't "treatment hop" if a line doesn't live up to its advertising right away. Give it a good six months to see how—or if—it changes your skin. Miracles don't happen in a month. Of course, if your skin shows any adverse reactions, discontinue use immediately.

You don't need to worry about mixing up makeup lines. It's perfectly fine to use a base from one place, a blusher from another. The formulations are all pretty standard.

Your Skin Type

The treatment products, and eventually the makeup, you select should be formulated specifically for your skin type. Before you can choose the products that will be of maximum benefit, you need to determine your skin's characteristics. And it's not so complicated. Basically, either skin is a problem to maintain or it is not. All skin types, at one time or another, can share a combination of characteristics. And when you add the complications of climate, diet, air-conditioning, central heating, seasonal changes, and emotional changes, you'll understand why your skin can develop different problems almost from moment to moment! Here's how to identify which classification most applies.

First, pull your hair back from your face with a hair band or scarf. Stand so that a good, strong light strikes your face evenly. Hold a mirror up to your well-cleansed face (allowing time for your skin to normalize after cleansing), and look for obvious clues to your skin's personality: dry patches, flaking, shiny spots, tiny red blood vessels showing close to the skin, fine lines, red or white splotches, dull complexion, enlarged pores, blackheads.

Next, stretch your face into a wide grimace. Note if it feels supple or tight. Relax your face and check to see if grimace lines remain. Now press your skin gently with your fingertips. Does it feel soft or rough? Does it spring back to the touch? Are there slippery patches, sticky spots?

Jot down these general characteristics, then look for the type they represent.

No-Problem Skin

No-problem skin is perfectly hydrated in the depths and on the surface. The protective oily barrier is sufficient to keep the skin soft and to retain the moisture underneath without making the skin appear shiny or feel sticky. When the underlying cells are properly "plump" with water, the skin has a smooth, even surface. This reflects the light and gives the complexion a fresh, healthy glow. Although no-problem skin can have its share of difficulties and can also react adversely to environmental conditions, it is essentially healthy in its appearance and responsive to proper attention. Care for it well, and you will have no-problem skin for life.

Some essentially no-problem skin is very fine. The epidermal layer is thin and contains less moisture than normal. This type of skin often peels, even with adequate deep hydration, and may develop fine wrinkles or flaky patches. It reacts easily to sun, cold, wind, and dust, and to chemicals like those in soaps and detergents or to products containing alcohol. The difference between this skin type and a true dry-skin condition is in the firmness and elasticity of the supporting tissues. Spot-moisturizing only the driest areas is effective treatment. Select an oil-based moisturizer to provide an emollient shield that will keep the skin's fluids hydrating the surface.

Another type of essentially no-problem skin has a thicker epidermal layer. The skin tends to retain moisture well on the surface, but the hydration of the deeper dermal layer may be insufficient. Although the skin is smooth and soft in appearance, there is a good chance it will lose its firmness and elas-ticity. When tissues under the skin begin to sag, lines are sure to appear. Only exercise can improve the circulation to the dermal layer and actually make thinning skin thicker.

HOW TO CARE FOR NO-PROBLEM SKIN

- Cleanse gently twice a day with a cleansing cream or lotion. Do not use soaps, detergent-based products, or abrasive cleansers.

- Follow every cleansing with a mild freshener to keep pores tight and to remove traces of cleanser clinging to the skin. Use an astringent with a low alcohol content.

- Avoid direct heat on the face—including that from blow dryers!

- Always use a mild, oil-based moisturizer under makeup to help retain surface moisture.

- Use a night cream on rough, dry patches when they occur.

- Guard against the drying, aging effects of the sun by using makeup products that contain a sunscreen. Remember that in addition to being dangerous, ultraviolet rays can damage collagen and thus reduce the skin's natural means of support.

- Once every two weeks, stimulate the circulation and smooth the surface of the skin by using a nondrying mask.

Dry Skin

Dehydrated skin is problem skin. Where once there was moisture, flaky or scaly patches appear. Tautness replaces suppleness. A soft, smooth complexion turns rough, uneven, even itchy. The telltale signs: dry white patches, red spots, tiny red veins (especially in the winter), a dull-looking complexion, thin lines around the eyes and mouth. It is a myth that dry skin does not produce oil; it does. But the amount produced is insufficient to retain an adequate amount of moisture in the epidermis. This "hydration filter" diminishes through a number of factors: aging, climate, sun abuse, central heating, use of detergent-based cleansers, metabolic changes, tiredness, stress, and infections or other illnesses that affect the production of sebum.

In short, dehydration of the outer surface of the skin is a condition we tend to bring on ourselves, depriving our skin of its natural protective shield and allowing precious cell moisture levels to drop. To undo the harm, dry skin must be handled with care. Think of your face as FRAGILE, and follow the cleansing and moisturizing techniques outlined below.

HOW TO CARE FOR DRY SKIN

- Avoid the use of tap water when cleansing; the deposits are too drying on the skin. And never, ever use hot water. To freshen your face, use only mineral water. Never use a washcloth—a rough texture can irritate. Wake up with a spray of mineral water misted on with a plant sprayer, and lightly pat dry.

- Use nondetergent, neutral-pH products to cleanse your skin—no soap! And always touch your face gently. Double-cleanse with a cream, leaving a light, thin trace of it on the skin after the second cleansing.

- Nourish and soften skin with an under-makeup moisturizer—every day. Use foundations with an oil base.

- If you don't have a good, strong moisturizer on your face on a cold, windy winter day, don't go out! Cold will cause any moisture your skin has to evaporate, and the wind will just accelerate the process.

- Stay out of overheated rooms; avoid sudden changes in temperature; protect yourself from wind and sun. Remember, your face is FRAGILE.

- At night, use a very creamy cleanser or oil (baby oil is perfectly all right). Remove residue with a spray of mineral water. Follow up with a night cream applied at least a half-hour before retiring. If you lie down immediately after applying cream, it will "puff-up" delicate tissues around the eyes.

- Use an antiwrinkle cream mask twice a month—but not if your skin is red, rough, or irritated.

Oily Skin

If dehydrated skin requires its share of tender loving care, oily skin needs even more attention. More than any other, this type of skin reflects a true imbalance. And, underneath all the apparent problems, oily skin can be dehydrated. If it has been badly treated with strong, alcoholic toners or exposed to the sun too long, it can dehydrate and still be oily—the worst of both worlds!

The characteristics of oily skin are easy to spot. Look for shine on nose, forehead, chin. Watch for dilated pores, a thick grain, a poorly elastic, nonresistant surface. This change in texture is what distinguishes a truly oily skin condition from an essentially normal skin that happens to have oily patches.

The worst thing you can do for skin of this nature is to go at it too aggressively. If your oil glands are overactive, you're not going to stop them by anything you do to the surface of the skin; all you will succeed in doing is damaging your skin. True care of this condition starts from within. You must limit the intake of all foods that stimulate the sebaceous glands and restrict the amount of alcohol in your diet. Watch your intake of foods with a high iodine content and those containing hormones or hormonelike substances (kelp, beef liver, asparagus, milk, wheat germ, potato and tortilla chips, highly salted processed foods, peanut oil, corn oil, and wheat germ oil). Proper cleansing and care will take it from there.

HOW TO CARE FOR OILY SKIN

- Choose your cleanser with care. Avoid heavy cleansing creams. Try an antibacterial cleansing lotion or a lightly medicated soap, and use it in combination with a water rich in minerals, not tap water.

- When cleansing, massage your face well with your fingertips, using an upward and outward motion. Be careful not to rub soap into the skin; it can clog pores.

- Cleanse your face thoroughly two or three times a day, but avoid hard scrubbing and hot water. Energetic friction is the enemy of oily skin. You don't want to strip away all your natural oils.

- Follow morning cleansing with an astringent; use a milder toner in the evening. Strong astringents will do more harm than good, stimulating an overproduction of oil.

- Before applying makeup (select water-based products only), use an antiseptic day cream with active ingredients that diminish sebaceous secretions. Look for benzyl peroxide in the list of active ingredients.

- Use a light antiseptic night cream from time to time if you wish, and apply a clarifying mask one or two times a week.

- Have your face professionally deep-cleansed once every two months.

To Tone or Not to Tone?

All freshly cleansed skin requires some form of finishing to give it a smooth, lively appearance and to remove any traces of cleanser. The question is not whether to tone but which type of toner to use on your skin. And what's the difference, anyway, between a toner, a freshener, an astringent, and a clarifying lotion?

First of all, they are all toners and will refresh the skin after cleansing. What distinguishes them, primarily, is their ratio of water to alcohol. (*Note:* Many manufacturers use these terms interchangeably, so check the ingredients listing for the water/alcohol content to be sure.)

Skin Fresheners have more water than alcohol. They are the mildest toners and will remove cleanser residue. Some fresheners contain certain irritating ingredients, however, such as sugar, fragrance, and rosewater.

Astringents rely on alcohol to remove traces of dirt. Many contain antibacterial agents as well.

Clarifying Lotions are the strongest types of toners, containing more alcohol than water, and usually have other chemical agents to remove the top layer of dead skin.

Moisturizing: A Must

Both no-problem skin and problem skin can benefit from proper moisturizing. But don't for a moment think that a moisturizer is what *supplies* the moisture; in spite of its name, it really doesn't. A moisturizer's main job is to provide an additional protective shield to keep the moisture that's there *there*. Of course, the water content in every moisturizer will help to replenish some surface moisture. But true hydration of the skin happens deep in its lower layers—where no moisturizer can penetrate.

A good moisturizer will stay on top of the skin, not sink in (although night creams are heavier and go deeper). And the more oil a moisturizer has, the more effective it will be in preventing the escape of moisture from the surface of the skin. If your skin has too much oil, naturally you should select a moisturizer with more water than oil. It will be lighter and less greasy. All things being equal, however, your skin will benefit more from a moisturizer that lists oil before water in its ingredients. Learn to recognize oil as an ingredient, no matter what it may be called. Lanolin, collagen, jojoba, aloe, mineral oil, turtle oil, mink oil, and swan oil are just a few of its disguises.

If you don't choose the right moisturizer for your skin type, and it is not nourishing your skin properly, your makeup will tend to fade quickly. If your moisturizer doesn't stay on top of your skin, your makeup will disappear with it! Makeup that changes color is another sign that something is going wrong. But the problem is not with your makeup—it's with your moisturizer. Again, it's been badly chosen for your skin type. Best to throw it out and try a new product.

Take advantage of the moments you must spend moisturizing your skin by turning them into minimassage sessions. One trick is to put the dab of moisturizer on the *back* of one of your hands so you can free both hands for a self-massage. Start at the base of the neck, stroking upward, one hand after the other. Pat underneath your chin, then continue lightly stroking upward and outward on your face. Use your knuckles along the sides of your nose. Use a press/release technique across your forehead and eyebrow ridge. Follow this same upward-stroking procedure when you are taking your makeup off. Always make it a light massage. Your face will feel much better every time you touch it!

Taking Makeup Off

Proper skin care is a process that continues throughout the day—from the soothing awakening of skin in the morning, through the gentle application of makeup, to the final cleansing at night. Although makeup can act as a protective barrier by day, shielding the face from airborne dirt and moisture-robbing winds, by night makeup can turn against the skin. If not thoroughly and properly removed, it can trap the grime of the day on the face, clogging pores and causing trouble!

Take your time with makeup removal, and your skin will be invigorated. Make it a habit, and it won't be a complicated procedure at all. One general tip: Make every movement in a direction opposite to the way wrinkles form. Wipe across vertical lines; smooth up and across horizontal lines. Here's the whole process.

1. Get Ready
Have six to eight cotton pads ready and waiting. Wet each one under the tap, and press the water out between your fingers.

2. Cleanse Eyes
Always start with the eyes—one at a time. Close one eye, look with the other. Cleanse the first eye completely before you begin the second one. Apply eye makeup remover to a cotton pad. Wipe the pad from the brow downward over your closed lid to the base of your lashes. Repeat several times until the entire lid is clean. Open your eye. Clean the

residue left under the lower lashes by bringing the pad from the outside to the inside corner of the eye and wiping off the remaining makeup.

3. Blot
Immediately blot the eye area with a tissue to remove all traces of oily remover.

4. Repeat
Start on the other eye with a clean cotton pad. Use as many cotton pads as you need to remove every trace of makeup. Blot with a tissue when done. Remember to respect the skin around the eye—it is extremely fragile. Never pull, never press.

5. Next, Throat and Jawline
Apply cleansing cream to another clean cotton pad. If you are right-handed, start at the left side of your neck, just above the collarbone, and stroke the pad upward to the jawline. Repeat in six side-by-side strokes. Do the same on the right side of your neck. Reverse the order if you are left-handed.

6. Stroke Across Jaw and Cheek
Saturate a fresh cotton pad with cleansing cream. Begin at the center of your chin, follow your jawline to the left, and lift the pad at your ear. Repeat the same wiping movement from the left corner of your nose to your ear. Then sweep the pad upward, starting below the left corner of your mouth and ending at the corner of the left eye. Continue to stroke underneath the eye, taking the pad out to the temple. Repeat the same procedure on the right side of your face.

7. Clean the Forehead
Take the pad from the left temple across to the right temple in six even strokes.

8. Pay Extra Attention to the Nose
Wipe the pad down the bridge of the nose (the only spot on your face where you should use a downward movement), and rotate the cotton pad carefully around the nostrils.

9. Remove Lipstick
Draw a fresh pad across the lips from the left side of the mouth to the right, turning it over, and bringing it back from the right side of the mouth to the left. Blot cleansing cream off with a tissue.

10. Blot
Lift excess cream off the entire face, lightly pressing with a tissue. If you wear a lot of makeup, repeat the *entire* process once more.

11. Cleanse as Usual
Follow the normal cleansing routine for your skin type described earlier in this chapter, finishing up with a toner or an astringent.

Special Care: Skin Care for Changing Seasons

Proper skin care doesn't exist in a vacuum. The weather constantly affects all exposed areas. And nothing is more exposed to dry heat, sticky humidity, cold wind, and the sun's damaging rays than your face. So you must take the calendar into account when you plan your skin-care regimen. Depending on the season and the weather, you must moisturize differently, protect differently, and use your beauty time differently. What works for you in summer may be disastrous when the first chill winds blow. And you may overprotect your skin on those winter days when there's more moisture in the air. Here's a four-season plan to keep your skin glowing all year through!

Fall

Autumn is the time to settle your skin down after summer sun, sweat, salt water, and chlorine have done their damage. Slough off dead cells with a professional facial. Revitalize skin with masks and rejuvenating creams. Your skin has already suffered too much and needs a lot of tender care. If your skin is normal-to-dry, switch to an oil-based moisturizer and use a moisturizing makeup.

Winter

In the winter concentrate on protecting your skin and lips. Use heavier, oilier moisturizing products than you normally use. Apply a body moisturizer after every shower or bath. Keep lips soft with petroleum jelly at night, a lip balm with sunscreen by day. Use lipsticks with built-in moisturizers and conditioners.

Spring

Perk up winter-weary skin with a good facial in the spring. Begin to lighten up on your moisturizer. It can still be oil-based if you like, but not as heavy or as oily as winter's. Go into the sun gradually. Don't ruin your complexion on the first warm day. You'll have all summer to cultivate a healthy "glow."

Summer

Summer means protecting your face and lips from too much sun. In addition to aging your skin, an overly dark tan detracts from a beautiful, feminine look—and it competes with any color you put on your face. Keep skin well moisturized, but switch to a lighter, water-based product. Be sure to wear a special lip sunscreen for any prolonged exposure to the sun.

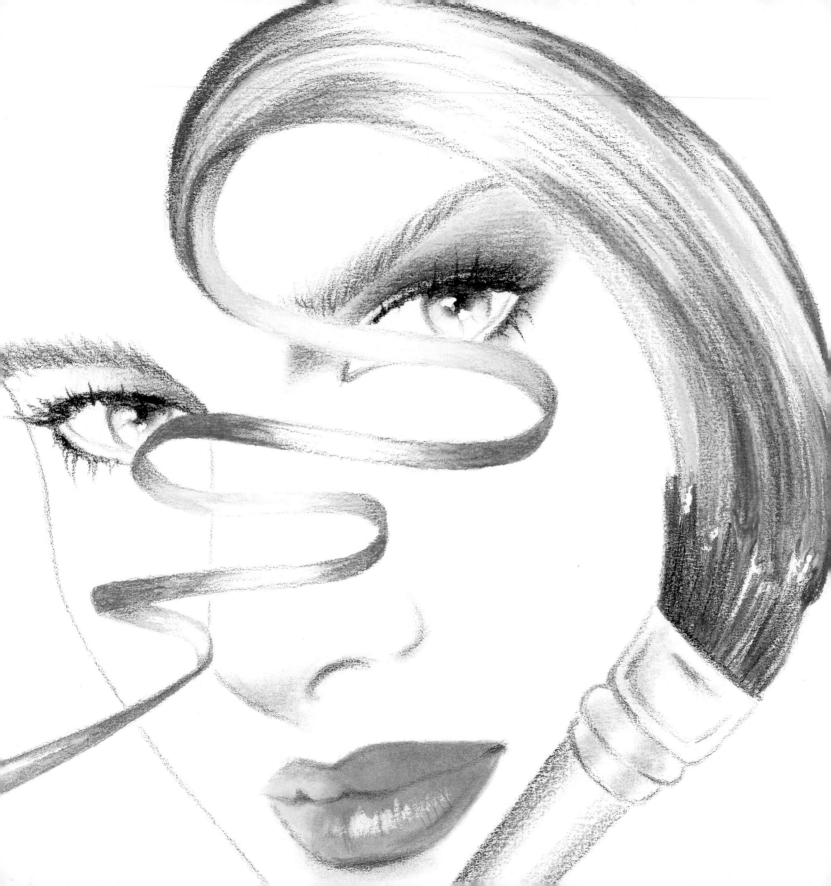

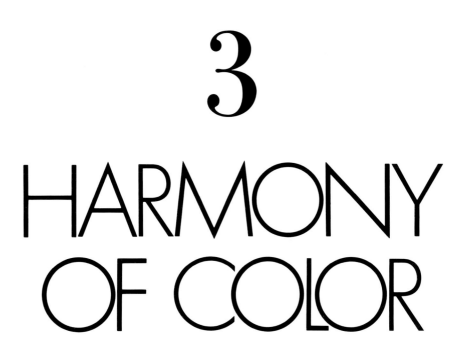

3
HARMONY OF COLOR

Every woman is entitled to more adventure in her beauty.
Setting a limit on the colors she should wear denies her possibilities.

The very lifeblood of the cosmetics industry is the creation of new shades, new excitement, season after season. What the industry ends up creating for a lot of women is confusion. If you think the palettes change just when you've decided on your favorite shades, you're not alone. That's why many women refuse to try new colors: they find one or two "old friends" and stick with them.

Don't let this happen to you. If you wear one palette all the time, you'll be casting your face in stone. You'll show no spontaneity, no spark. You'll lack the flexibility to adapt to the latest fashion looks. And you may be settling for something far less than your maximum attractiveness. You'll be limiting your options when it comes to what you want to wear and the way you want to look. If you typecast yourself, you'll fall into a color trap.

If you want the freedom to wear whatever colors you choose—and every woman should have that freedom—you need to know how to bring your personal coloring (complexion tone, eye color, and hair color) into harmonious balance with the colors you wish to wear. And it's not that difficult to do. You need first to identify your own complexion undertone, then learn how to adapt it to any color family. And you need to select a coordinated palette of tones—a harmony of color—within the color family you wish to wear.

A total harmony of color includes your base shade, your eye makeup (shadows, liners, and mascara), and your cheek and lip colors. When these blend with both your natural coloring and your clothing, you have created a harmony of color.

There are two basic palettes from which to select a harmony of color: a blue range and a yellow range. Why these two? Because all harmonies start with your basic complexion tone. Fair or dark, you will have a complexion with an underlying blue cast or a yellow cast. If you add a tan, you will have to heighten the shades you normally use and select from a third color range: the tan tone palette.

Your Natural Colors

It is important to be open to the new colors of each season, but you should also know how to select from the season's offerings with confidence. That's where understanding your own coloration comes into play. There are three different aspects of your coloring to consider, and each influences the makeup you select to wear at any given time. Let's take them one by one.

Hair Color

Of course hair color can change, but generally this important frame for your face is constant over a period of time. You must select your makeup accordingly. More than any other feature, your hair color will influence the touches of color you add to your face, especially the lip shades. As a general rule, hair and lip shades should balance each other. The lighter the hair, the lighter the lips. The darker the hair, the darker the lips. Vivid lips in contrast to pale blonde or gray hair look too startling. Pale lips framed by dark hair tend to disappear.

Complexion Tone

To determine your skin's predominant undertone, check the back of your wrist (find a spot that hasn't been exposed to the sun). A bluish-tinged complexion may have veins close to the surface or appear slightly pink to ruddy. A complexion with predominantly yellow undertones will appear more beige, slightly yellow to olive.

Eye Color

Unless you have a wardrobe of tinted contacts, your eye color is another constant, and certain tones will work best with their color. These are the Corresponding Shadow Colors. You would select them if you are wearing shades in the same color family as your eyes (see chart opposite). If not, you'll learn how to "neutralize" your natural eye color to wear any eye shadow shade you want in the following pages.

EYE COLOR	CORRESPONDING SHADOW COLORS
Blue, gray	Blue, pink, mauve, violet, pink/beige, gray, slate, burgundy
Brown, hazel	Yellow, beige, taupe, brown, gray, peach, apricot
Green	Yellow/green, lime, olive, coral, peach, brown, yellow/beige

Working with Your Natural Colors

The shades you select to wear on your eyes, cheeks, and lips at any given time are what give your face a general harmony of color. These touches of color are influenced by (1) your general complexion tone and (2) the color of your clothing. Here's how it works.

Best Makeup Shades

The most important thing to remember when adding touches of color to your makeup is to keep the palette consistent all the way through. That is absolutely essential if you don't want your face to suddenly go "tilt." If you are coordinating a blue/pink harmony of color, don't switch to a bright copper lipstick midway through. Go with mauve or wine. If you're coordinating a beautiful peachy-apricot palette, don't resort to blue eye shadow

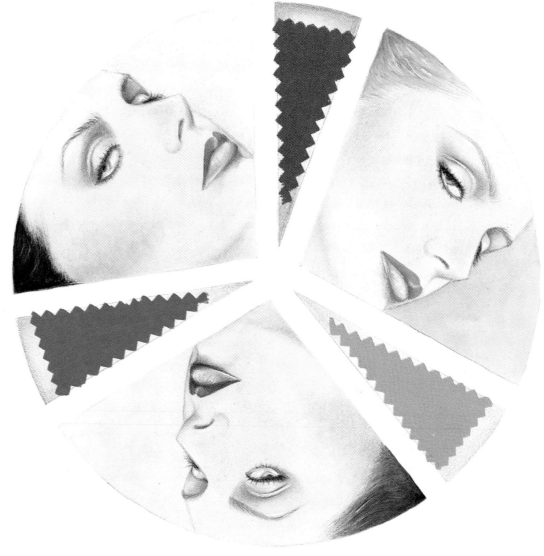

If you have tawny or yellow undertones to your complexion, you'd select a yellow/beige palette, starting with a beige/ivory base, a tawny or coral blush, apricot/peach lip color, and eye shadows in the beige/taupe/brown/ olive/peach family. ▼

◀ If you have a blue undertone to your complexion, the blue/pink palette is for you. You might begin with a pinky-beige base. You could select a pink or burgundy blush, pink or bluish-red lip color, and eye shadows in the mauve/violet/pink/blue range. If you have blue eyes, you may find it more flattering to stick with blue/slate shadows. Brown eyes may be prettier with mauve/burgundy colors. And green eyes would be softer with violet/ purple shades.

because you have blue eyes. In spite of what you think, it won't enhance them. They'll look like strangers with the rest of your makeup. Try gray closest to your eye, then highlight with a soft peach. It is much more flattering to stay with one coordinated color palette. The three Harmony of Color charts that follow give you directions for eye, lip, and cheek colors that are compatible with your natural coloring.

Color of Clothing

Your choice of clothing is where your palette really crystallizes. It's such an important consideration that you should never, ever begin your makeup without knowing what you are going to put on. Too many women think what happens from the neck down has little or no relation to the face. But of course it does. Your clothing puts the most color right next to your skin; it must be compatible with the colors on your face. So essential is the harmony between makeup and wardrobe colors that I often advise women to look in their closets, determine the most dominant color in their wardrobe, and select their makeup shades around this color. Makeup is beautiful only when it continues the overall color impact.

The swatches of fabric shown with each color chart suggest the wardrobe colors that are most attractive with each palette: blue/burgundy/violet/pink for a blue/toned complexion; brown/gold/rust/beige for a yellow-toned complexion.

For tan or darker skins, you'd select touches of color from the tan tone palette, upping blusher and lip colors to copper or red and going to stronger shades (not brighter or lighter ones) for eye shadows. ▼

Working Around Your Natural Colors

What if you want to wear colors from one palette and your natural coloring is better with another? You have to know how to make your natural coloring compatible with the shades you choose to wear.

Correct Noticeable Tones

Your natural complexion undertone—blue, yellow, or tan—doesn't lock you into one makeup palette for life! Years ago, choosing the wrong color of base for your complexion would have created a very artificial look. Today, thanks to the vast variety of sheer tints on the market, it is possible to change your complexion tone with the mere application of a pink/beige base, a yellow/ivory base, or an earth/sienna bronzer and then select corresponding touches of color to complete the palette.

Complexions that have noticeable secondary tones may need more serious correction before they can take on a blue/pink, yellow/beige, or tan/red palette. You may be obviously pale or highly ruddy, slightly gray, yellow, or green. Or you may have only splotches where the color goes wrong (red veins under the eyes, tiny blue lines around the nose, darker areas on the forehead).

The point is to correct your complexion tone only if it is really noticeable—and only *where* it is noticeable. Do not cover your entire face with a colored mask. Instead, correct any trouble zones with color-tinted moisturizers or sheer washes of color. I don't recommend the corrective powder shades on the market if you're just beginning to experiment. They are more difficult to work with, since the powder sits on top of the skin and can be more noticeable. Liquid colors can be applied under your normal base or blended softly over it. Even worn alone, these sheer complexion correctors will neutralize a noticeable tone so that you can begin to build whatever palette you wish.

Choose the proper corrective tint to counteract any pronounced coloration in your skin tone.

Trouble Tone	Corrective Tint	Effect
Too yellow	Apricot	Warms sallowness; enhances a tan that is turning yellow
Too ruddy	Green	Tones down red
Too pale	Mauve	Enhances paleness and gives face a glow
Too blue/gray	Pink	Adds warmth

Neutralize Your Eyes

If you've got big blue eyes and are planning to wear a pink dress, nothing could be better. Both are in the same palette, so you would simply select eye shadow shades in your corresponding colors. If you have green eyes, however, you don't have to give the pink dress away, even if the best eye shadow shades for your coloring are in the yellow/green and peach tones. You can simply "neutralize" your natural eye color by rimming your lids with one of the intermediate tones listed below.

Intermediate Tones

Gray	Navy
Beige	Dark mauve
Black	Taupe
Brown (light to dark)	

You are now ready to add a color that would normally not be compatible with your eye color. To wear a blue/pink eye shadow, for instance, you would add a thin line of an intermediate tone like deep mauve at the lash line, *then* add the blue/pink color above the neutralized rim. This trick works any time you wish to wear a shadow that's not among your compatible shades. Simply rim the lid with one of the intermediate tones in a coordinating color. (You would not select a mauve tone, for instance, if you want to wear apricot; brown would be better.)

The next time you find yourself saying, "I could never wear _____ ," stop and think again. Maybe the color has never been wrong for you. Maybe your makeup has been wrong for the color. Sooner or later you're going to buy that gold coat or that magenta sweater, and now you know it's simply not a question of switching your lipstick to make it work. You know you've got to begin to build a harmony of color from the base up, compensating for your basic complexion tone if it's too far off, and continuing the palette with touches of color from the same family. If you don't limit yourself in the colors you select to work with, you'll be able to wear any clothing shade you want!

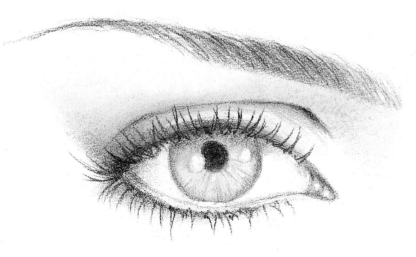

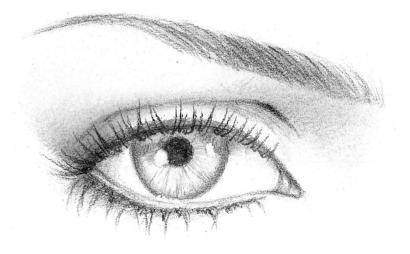

Gray Face Remedies

Too much makeup and too much fun the night before—or even a bout with the flu—can turn your face into a ghost of its former self. When you wake up to a gray face day, a minimum morning makeup won't do. You've got to give yourself a boost. But don't simply double up on your blusher; it will be all too obvious. The contrast against pale skin will make you look even more pallid. Try these instant perks instead:

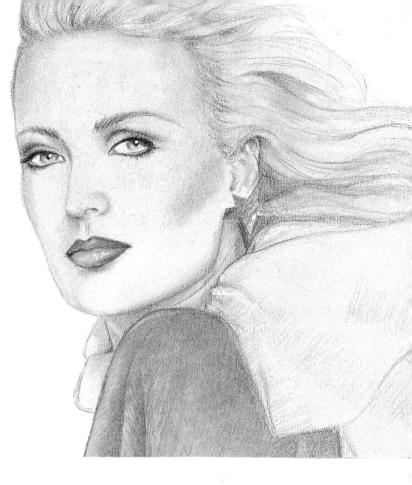

1. Rev Up Circulation
Work on your complexion first. Stimulate it with a massage as you cleanse, a brisk pat as you apply toner.

2. Apply Base and Blot
Use a light, transparent base—or a tinted moisturizer—with a pink touch.

3. Powder Over
Powder lightly—lightly! Top with a pink powder blush.

4. Avoid Eye Shadow
No blues, violets, or mauves. (After all, what color is an undereye circle?) Don't go near these tones today. You'll look tired by association! A simple layer of mascara and a bit of blusher on the browbone is enough.

5. Pick a Pretty Lip Color
Avoid lipstick with orange in it. It drains any pink right out of the complexion. Pink tones are better than peach; blued reds are better than browned reds. Shades of coral and cin-namon should be saved for another day. A very natural-looking rose or pink is your best bet. Avoid any color that's too bright. The rest of your face will pale by comparison.

6. Add Brightness
Think of color as a happy vitamin—but put it *near* your face, not on it. A yellow scarf or sweater (even if you normally wouldn't wear that color) or anything in the rose/fuchsia family will brighten your whole aspect.

7. Think Positive Thoughts
Look forward to the most agreeable part of the day. A positive thought should put some sparkle back into your eyes.

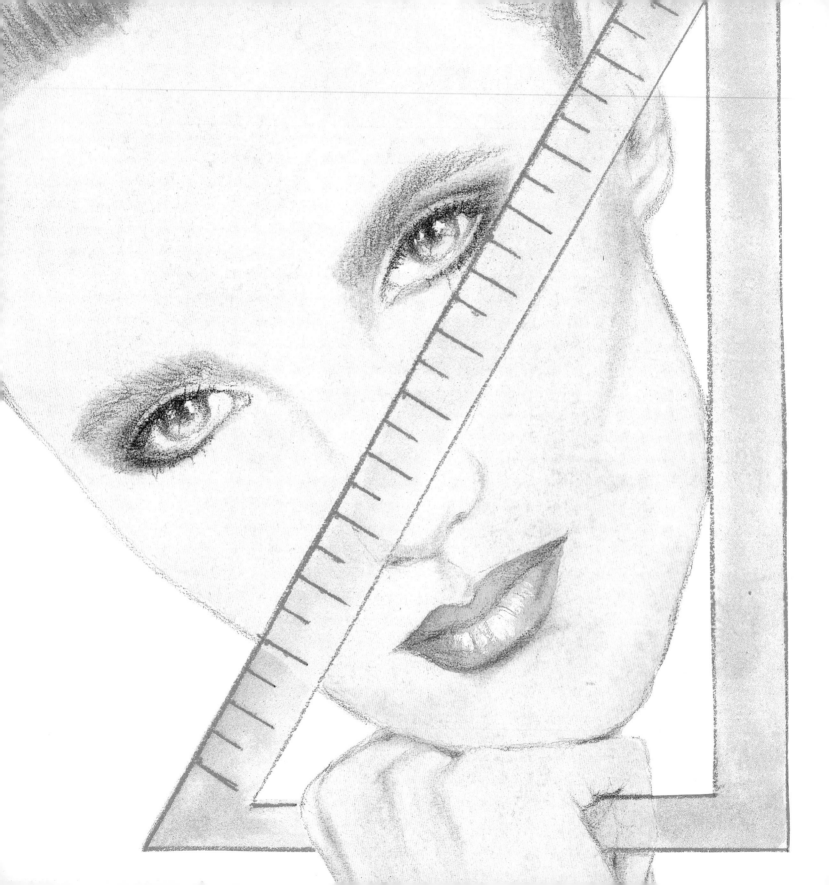

4
FORM OF FACE

Not all imperfections are to be shaded.
Sometimes they become a part of your beauty.

Nothing influences the placement of makeup so much as the form of your face. The basic structure of your facial bones, the arrangement of your features, the shadows and lights they create—all play a part in determining where, and how, you apply makeup.

When you think of the legendary beauties, you are more likely to remember the ones with distinctive facial characteristics. A squared chin, an impressive nose, surprising brows. You do not want to camouflage those features that give your face an individual, distinctive beauty. Yet you can learn to *balance* those features that are taking focus. The key is to remember that your beauty must be the sum of its parts. If any one characteristic takes over, it's to your best advantage to learn how to proportion it to your total image.

It is absolutely essential, then, to get a true reading of the form of your face. I am always surprised at the number of women who ask me what their facial shape is. Face shapes are not difficult to recognize, but you must be totally honest in your appraisal. There are many things you can do with makeup to give your face the shape you wish it had, but you must always start with the shape it does have.

The Basic Face Shapes

The best way to see the real bone structure of your face is first to pull all your hair back with a hair band or scarf. (The hair acts as a frame for the face, and it can mislead you.) Next, wash your face and apply a light cold cream over it. (Any trace of makeup may create a shape that simply isn't there.) Finally, position a strong light so that it reflects equally and evenly over the surface of your skin. Now look in the mirror. The light reflecting off the cream should tell you all you need to know. You'll see by the highlights and shadows what protrudes and what recedes. The essential bone structure should be clearer than it has ever been before. And you should be able to tell easily if your face appears to be more (1) oval, (2) round, (3) square, or (4) long. Don't look for triangles or hearts or diamond shapes. If your face does not fit into one of the four basic shapes, you may simply have a combination of two of the shapes. It is possible, for instance, to have a basically square face with an oval chin. Or a long face with a squared-off jawline.

Comparing the proportions of your facial features to those of the ideal oval face shape, at right, will give you some clues as to the shape of your own face. The oval, for example, is divided horizontally into thirds by the eyebrows and the bottom of the nose; the eyes are separated by a distance equalling the length of one eye. Now look at your own face. Is the distance from your nose to your chin longer than one-third of the total length of your face? If yes, chances are that your face is on the long side. Shorter? It may be somewhat round.

If you do have a combination face shape, it's not complicated to plan a makeup strategy. You simply do a combination makeup following the techniques that are right for each particular portion of the face. And the Face Finder at the end of this chapter lets you mix and match face shapes to find the makeup placement that's exactly right for you. For now, though, it is enough to know the basic shape of your face.

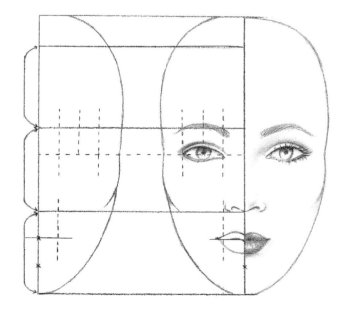

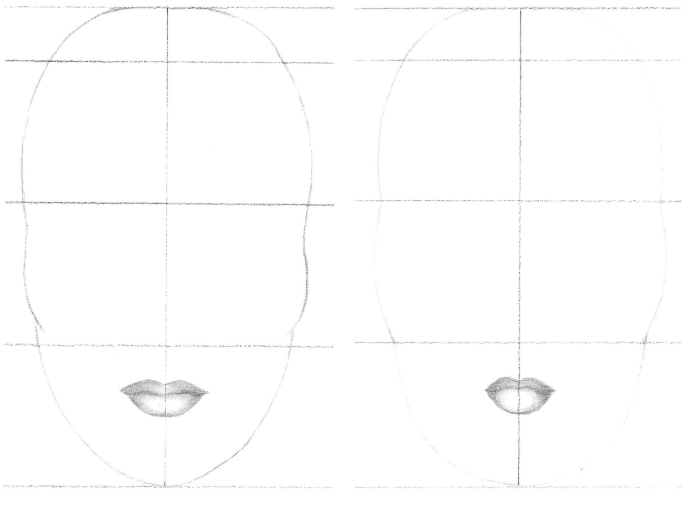

Oval ▲   Round ▲

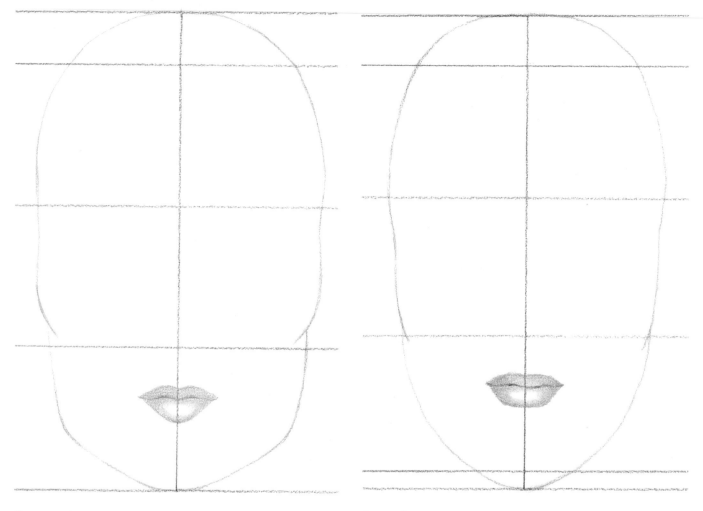

Square ▲

Long ▲

Understanding Dark and Light

Once you've identified the shape of your face, you can alter its shape relatively easily, if you wish, through makeup. You don't need to be a master artist to do so, but it is helpful to understand a few artistic principles before you begin to experiment.

Creating form is not so much a question of shades as it is of *shading*. Take all the color away, and form is merely a composition of dark and light. In artistic terms, this is called *chiaroscuro*—the distribution of light and shadow. The contours of your face provide the landscape where light and shadow alternately bring areas to attention or darken them into obscurity. Light accentuates, shadow recedes. It's as simple as that.

The best time to check for your own natural distribution of highlights and shadows is, again, when you have nothing on your face but a light cream and your hair is pulled away. Make sure the light strikes your face directly from the front. If you stand under the light, you'll have a horror show of shadows!

Once you see which areas are prominent and which are underemphasized, you are on your way to determining proper color selection. You will know to go with lighter shades— always—for areas you wish to bring out, and with darker tones—always—for areas you want to underplay.

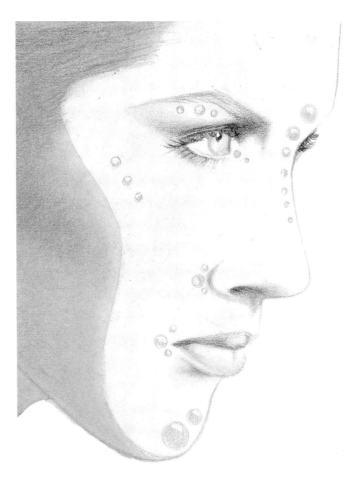

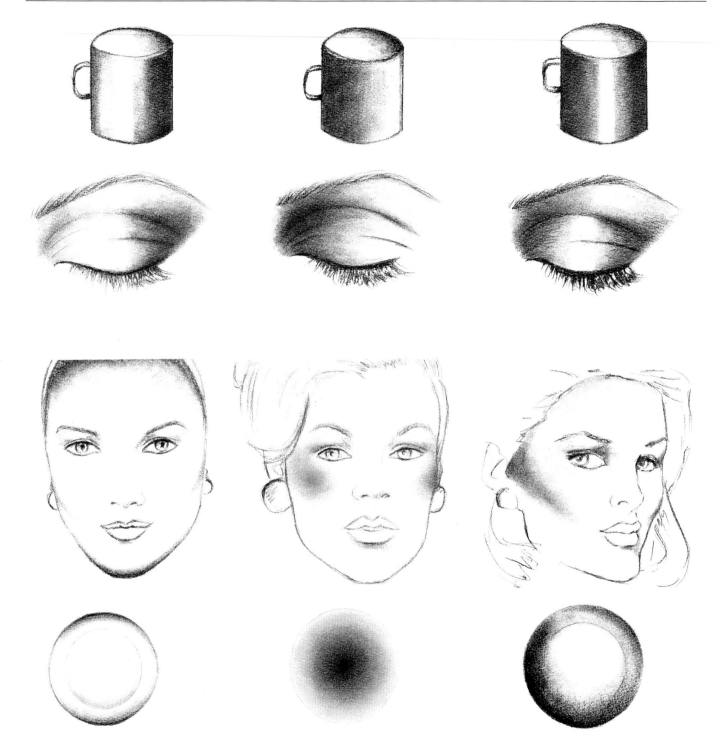

The Art of Blending

The selection and application of dark and light shades to the face is the next step in creating form. But this is where too many women run into trouble. The minute shading becomes obvious, it has defeated its own purpose. Attention becomes focused on the technique, not on the effect.

No makeup is beautiful unless it's blended. Color that just sits on the skin is too harsh, too unnatural. Obvious demarcations between colors look heavy-handed. You must always blend, every step along the way, whether you do it with a finger, a brush, a cotton ball, or all three.

It is very natural to put color on and "rub it in." You probably think you've been blending since the first moment you used makeup. But rubbing color in is about as far from proper blending as painting with a roller is from using a very fine brush. Blending is a special art that allows you to create light and dark *naturally*.

Blending is not simply a case of fading out a flat, constant color. Think of the way light strikes a curved surface, such as a cup or saucer. When a surface curves outward, you see a gradation of dark to light to dark. On the concave surface, it is just the reverse: light to dark to light. If you approach your face composition in terms of rounded areas and angles, following the "cup and saucer" school of blending, you will create a far more natural effect. You should never create a dark shadow without highlighting at least one side of it. And never use highlighting without adding a corresponding shadow to soften it. A wrinkle, for instance, needs to be lightened in its depth but shadowed along the pouchy area that surrounds it. A cheekbone, on the other hand, can be shadowed to create depth or hollowness, but the prominent bone should be highlighted at the same time. A beautiful eye shadow should accentuate the rounded surface of the lid. Instead of applying a uniform streak of color to the area, make the lid seem more curved by varying the intensity of the color or by using contrasting shades. You can go from dark to light to dark from the inner corner to the outer corner—or from light to dark to light from the browbone to the lashes.

It takes practice to perfect this kind of subtle shading, and you can start developing your technique by blending colors on a plain white sheet of paper. Stroke your finger across a cream blusher; then, by increasing the pressure of your fingertip halfway across the paper, take the streak from light to dark to light. Just underneath this line, reverse the effect. Start with a strong stroke and go from dark to light to dark by decreasing the pressure in the center of the stroke. Now compare the different optical effects the two lines give you. One will seem to curve in, the other out. Do the same with sponge applicators for eye shadow shading, and with brushes for blush shading. Create different shapes. Experiment with two or more eye shadow shades of different values to get the same light-to-dark and dark-to-light effects. Find out just what more pressure or less pressure can do. Once you can see the difference in front of you, you're ready to try your new techniques on your face.

Base Shading

The selection and application of dark and light shades to the face is the next step in creating form. This is where too many women run into trouble. The minute shading becomes obvious, it has defeated its own purpose. Attention becomes focused on the technique, not the effect. When it is done properly, base shading will make your face appear more balanced, better proportioned.

First, find the base-shading technique best suited to your face shape to bring it as close to the perfect oval as possible, without narrowing it too much. The effect you want is to bring out the maximum area on which to apply makeup; don't overshade the sides. To do this, you must begin with correctly shaped brows, using the arch as a point of measurement (see page 56 for brow shaping hints).

To determine what is to be shaded, bisect

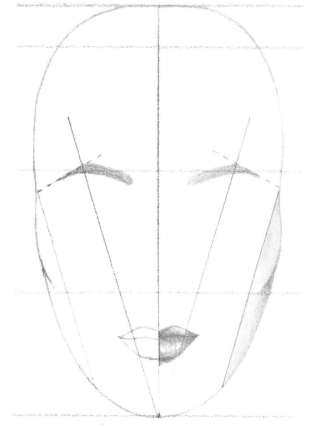

Oval
Because the oval is the ideal face shape, no special base-shading techniques necessary. ▲

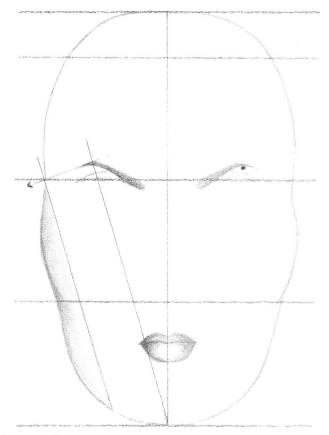

Round
Use a half shade darker in triangles from cheekbones to chin. ▲

your face vertically from chin to forehead. From the point of your chin, draw an imaginary line up to the inner arch of your eyebrow. From this point, continue the descending line of your brow out to your temple. Finally, draw a second imaginary line from your temple to jawline, running exactly parallel to the first line. Anything that falls outside this second line should be shaded.

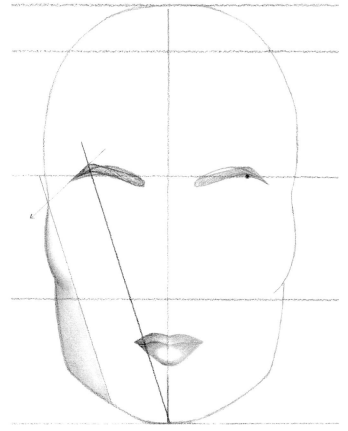

Square

Since you have a lot of shading to do, use two different shades of base. It will look far more natural than if you used a browned correcting shade or a blusher. Use triangles of the darker base from your hairline to your temples, tapering off right at the top edge of your cheekbone. Start your jawline shading just below the cheekbone, using inverted triangles of color that reach their widest point from jawline to chin. ▲

Long

Apply base in a triangle of color, with the widest part starting at the temples and the point ending at the chin. Then use a second, lighter shade to form two inverted triangles at the sides of the face, with the widest part going through the cheeks to the jawline. ▲

The Face Finder: Makeup Strategies for the Four Basic Face Shapes

Different faces require different makeup placement techniques to bring their features into perfect balance. If your face shape is a combination (for instance, a square forehead with an oval chin), you'll have to borrow placement techniques from more than one shape. Refer again to your face shape on page 40. Simply by cutting the next four pages on the dotted lines, you can mix and match until you find the precise shape of your face and the perfect makeup placement for each facial area. Once you've perfected the makeup placement for your face shape, refer to the correcting techniques on the following pages to fine-tune your makeup to your individual features.

EYEBROWS Slant them upward at the end to form little wings.

- -

Oval

You won't need corrective shaping techniques if you're lucky enough to have an oval face. Remember, this is the shape every other corrective makeup strategy tries to emulate. Simply follow the step-by-step makeup procedure outlined earlier in this chapter, keeping in mind that you want to accentuate the attractive roundness of your face.

EYE SHADOW Create an outward, almond shape with a sweep of color starting at the center of the lid and extending to just above the eye crease at the outside corner of the eye.

BLUSH Add a circle of blush just on the pillows of your cheeks, blending out.

- -

LIPS Keep them full.

CHIN Dab a dot of blush right in the center.

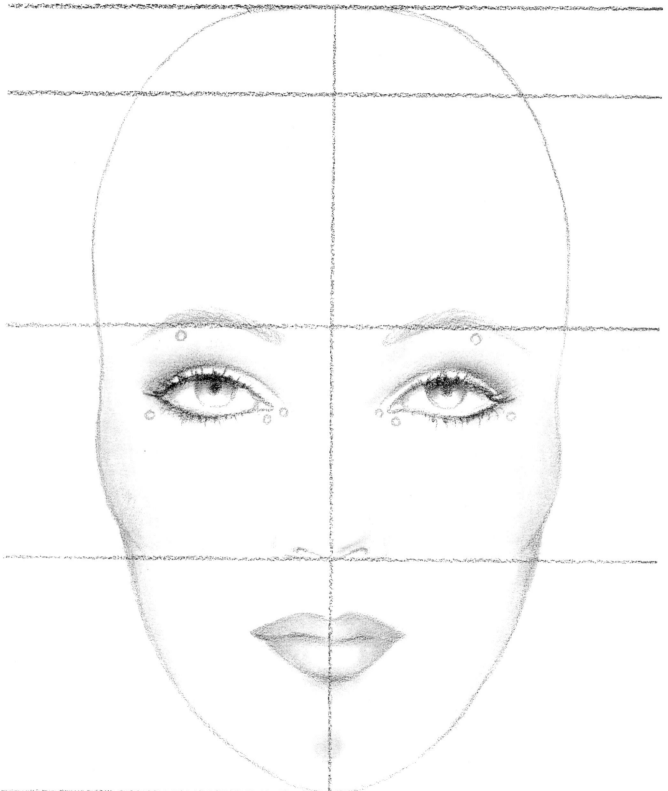

Round

Although some roundness does add prettiness to the face, you can have too much of a good thing. You'll need to practice subtle blending to make your face more oval in appearance. Think in terms of triangles and vertical lines.

EYEBROWS For this face shape *only*, keep brows short and rather high placed. (Longer, sweep-down brows turn a round face into a moon shape!)

EYE SHADOW Use high triangles of color on the outside corner of the eye, from lid to brow, to take attention away from rounded cheeks. Add highlight shadow in a diagonal sweep from the inside corner of the eye to the center of the browbone. Overlap the edges of color with the darker shade.

BLUSH Make a vertical sweep straight down the center of your cheek to contradict the roundness. Blend the bottom of the line upward and out toward your eye, creating a triangle. Add blusher at the right and left sides of the hairline, just above the temples.

LIPS Keep the mouth small and full. (A thin line makes a round face look like a "happy face" button!)

CHIN Add a triangle of blush to the chin.

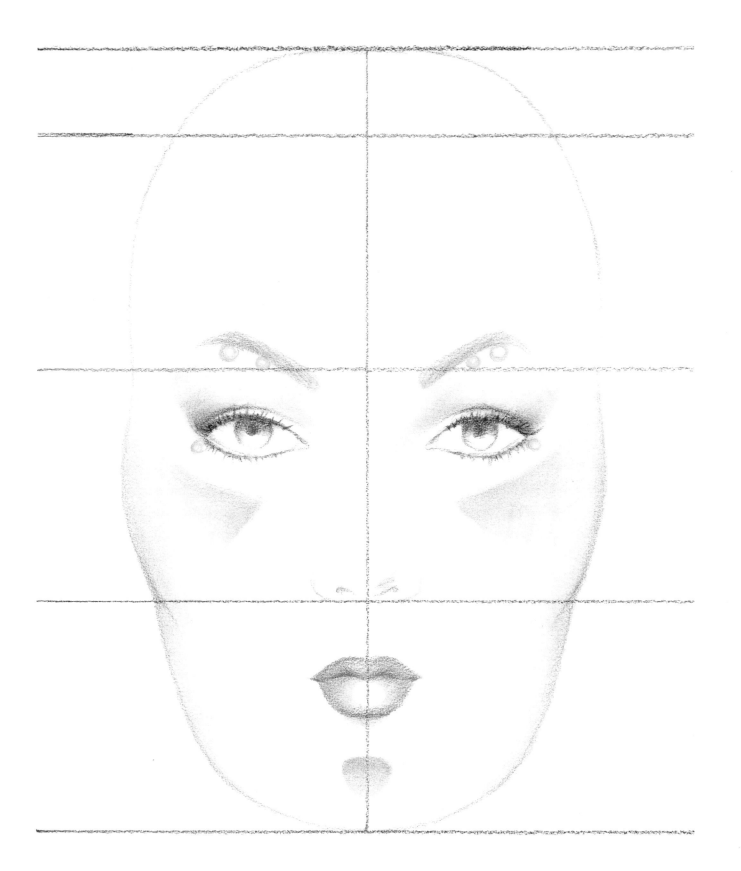

Square

If you have a strong jaw and a broad fore-head, you'll need to soften the basic structure of your face with shading. Remember to strive for an oval effect, and add contrasting angles with triangles of color.

EYEBROWS Add an angle by arching your brows directly in the center, in line with your pupils and cheekbones.

EYE SHADOW Start your highlighter just at the center of your lid. Sweep it straight up from the lash line to the center of your brow arch. Add a wedge of darker color from the center of your eyelid up and out to the end of your eyebrow. Overlap the edges of the two colors.

BLUSH Place blush just underneath the center of the cheekbone so that the accent is in the middle of the face; then blend out, angling the color up toward the ear.

LIPS Add another angle here to contrast with a wide jawline. Shape the lower lip into a slight triangle.

CHIN For another narrowing touch, add a triangle of blush to the center of the chin, tapering it to a point.

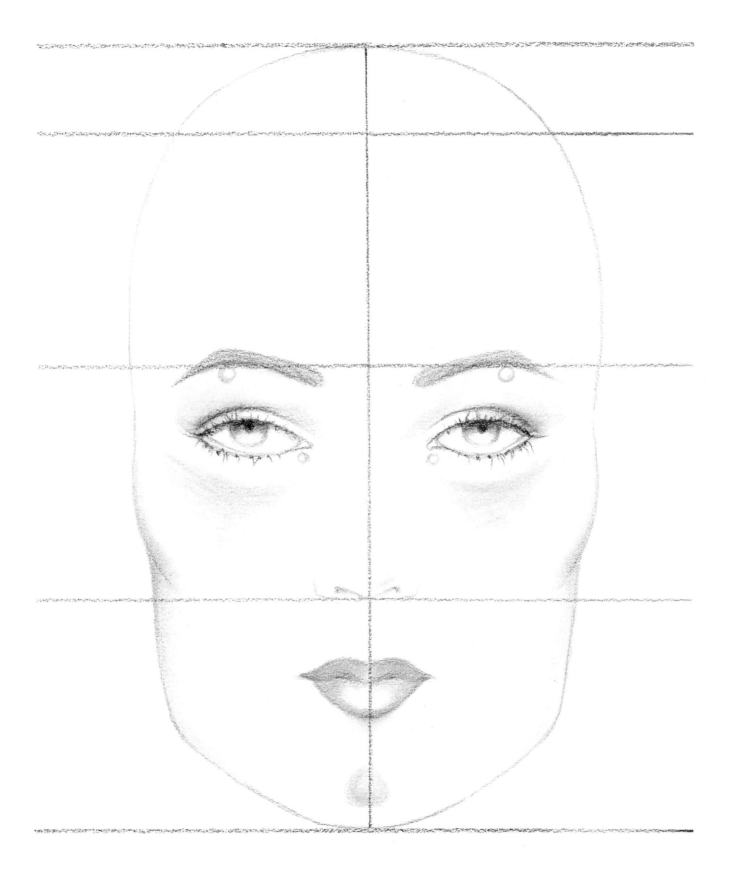

Long

Anything you can do to add horizontal lines to a long face will have a widening effect. Think in terms of sweeps of color—across the eyes, the cheeks, the mouth. Add an oval focal point by using a slightly darker base on the center of the face, a lighter base at the sides.

EYEBROWS Keep them as horizontal as possible, bending only a little at the end.

EYE SHADOW Use horizontal strokes of color, from the center of the eyelid out. Do not tilt color up at the outside corner of the eye. Color can reach up to the browbone, but it must be added in a straight (not an upswept) line.

BLUSH Add blush at the outside of the cheekbones, sweeping it across in a straight line. Corner it up to the temples. Never place blush in the center of the face. Add a horizontal sweep of blush across the hairline.

LIPS Outline lips to give them a horizontal line. Soften peaks on the upper lip and underplay the curve of the lower lip. Fill in with color all the way to the corners.

CHIN Shade under, not on, the chin with blusher extending the full length of the jawline.

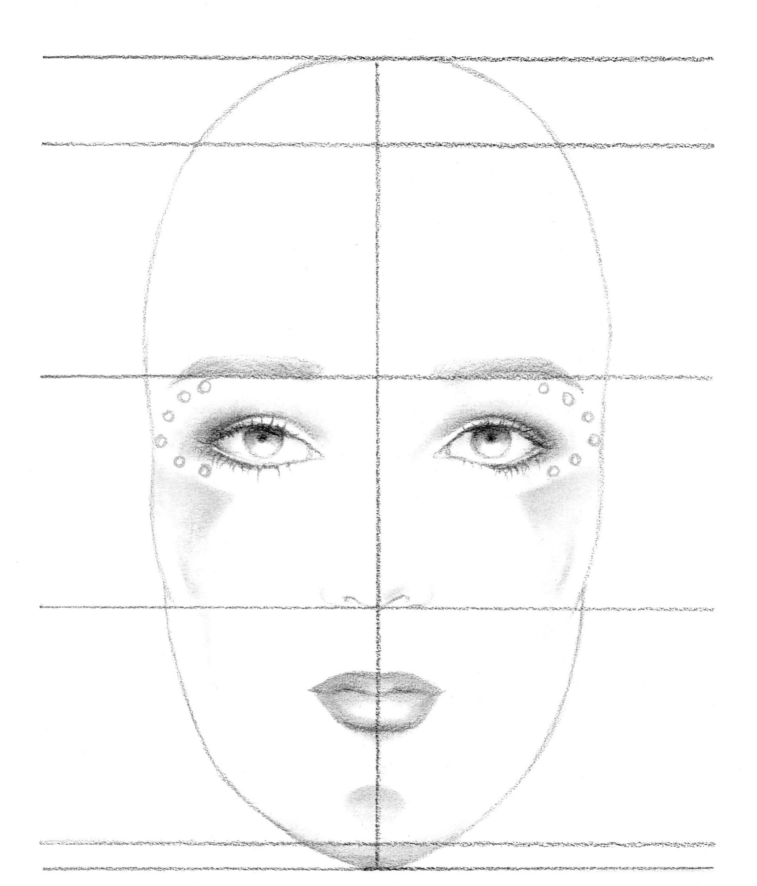

Correcting Techniques: Eyebrows

Today, every woman likes her eyebrows to look as natural as possible. But that isn't a license to forget them. They are too important to ignore.

Balance is the key attribute well-shaped eyebrows can give your face. They're your guidelines to perfect makeup placement and as such you must make sure their shape is right before you begin any other shaping or corrections with makeup. The length and arch of your brow will help you determine your base-shading technique, subtly influence the way your nose is perceived, and affect the placement of your eye makeup. There is nothing more disconcerting than eyebrows that end before the rest of your eye makeup does. You can't do elaborate extensions with a short brow or darker, dramatic makeup with a pale brow. It will look out of kilter. Properly shaped eyebrows will open up the center of your face, softening a prominent nose, strengthening a small one.

To plan the perfect eyebrow for you, study the architecture of your face. Each brow should follow the natural curve of the eye, of the lid, and of the line of the nose. It should plunge almost into the nose line, never stopping short of it. Feel along your browbone to the point where it begins to curve into the bridge of the nose. Draw a line straight up, from the inside corner of your eye to this point. Here is where your brow should begin. Next, hold an orange stick on the diagonal from the side of your nostril to the outside corner of your eye. The arc of the stick from the outside corner of the eye to the eyebrow will define the maximum length for your eyebrow without makeup. If you enlarge your eyes with shadows, pencils, or color you must always extend the line of your brow as well.

You can correct the shape of brows that don't follow this natural line by penciling in the ideal shape—with a very obvious outline—then removing any hairs that fall outside the line, plucking the hairs in the direction they grow.

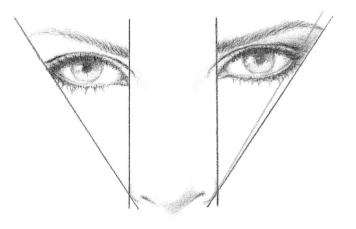

Some brows need more serious reshaping than just a light tweezing. You may need to combine selective tweezing techniques with penciled fill-ins. If you do use brow pencils, keep them subtle. You'll achieve a much more natural browline if you use a combination of two pencil colors. Use either gray and black or gray and brown to stroke in tiny lines. Never draw a horizontal line. Keep your strokes on the diagonal, going in the direction in which the hairs actually grow. Try the following techniques if your brows don't seem to fit your face.

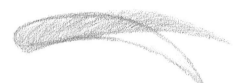

Too Droopy ▲
Pay attention to the extended line at the end, and tweeze away. The end of the brow should not go beyond the diagonal line from the nose to the outside corner of the eye. If you need to, tweeze under the center of the brow to form a natural, curved arch.

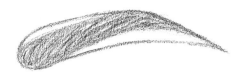

Too Thick ▲
Thin brows by tweezing random hairs—just enough so you can brush them neatly. If the shape that remains needs a more definitive arch, draw in the ideal shape with a pencil, then tweeze any hairs below this line.

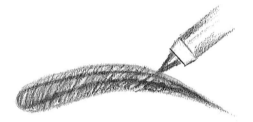

Too Thin ▲
Draw the ideal shape, adding width *both* above and below. Then fill in lines with short diagonal strokes, using two different colors. Start with the bottom line first, then add upward diagonal strokes from the bottom line to the top line.

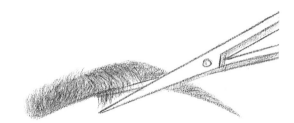

Too Bushy ▲
Comb all hairs straight down until your natural arch becomes apparent. With small manicure scissors, carefully trim the brushed-down brows, following the shape of the upper arch.

Too Arched ▲
Remove hairs only from the top and inside corner. Fill in just under the arch with tiny strokes.

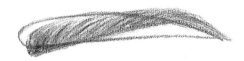

Too Straight ▲
Curve the browline toward the nose at the inside corner, and fill in that triangle. Extend the brow in a slight downward sweep at the end. Again, never go beyond the nose-to-eye diagonal line. Tweeze underneath the center of the brow to form a natural arch.

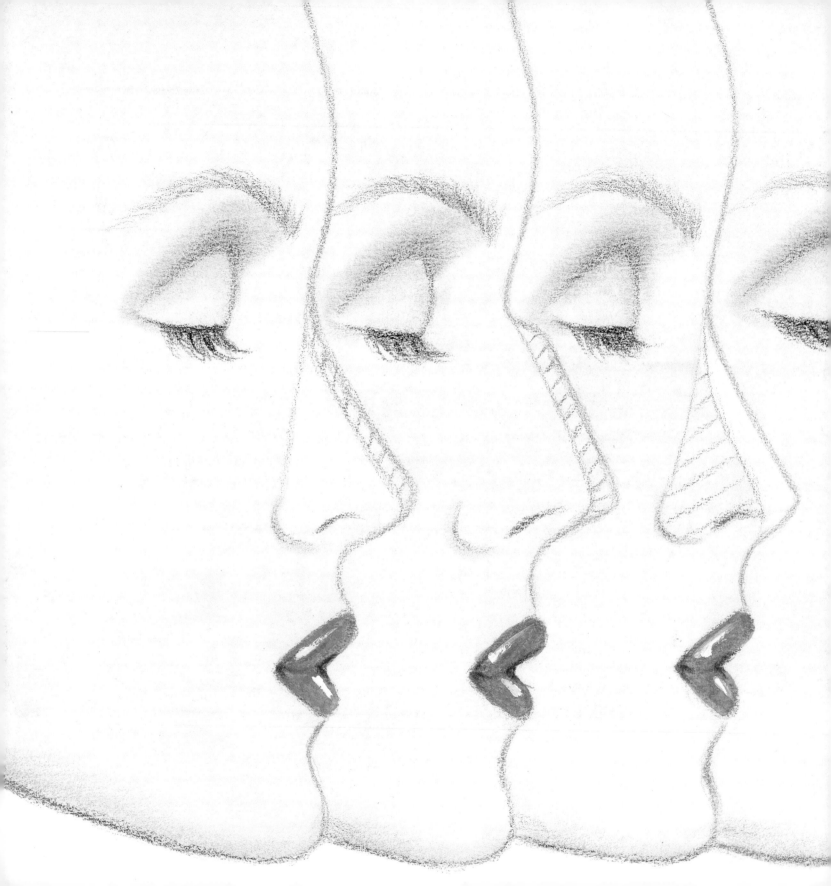

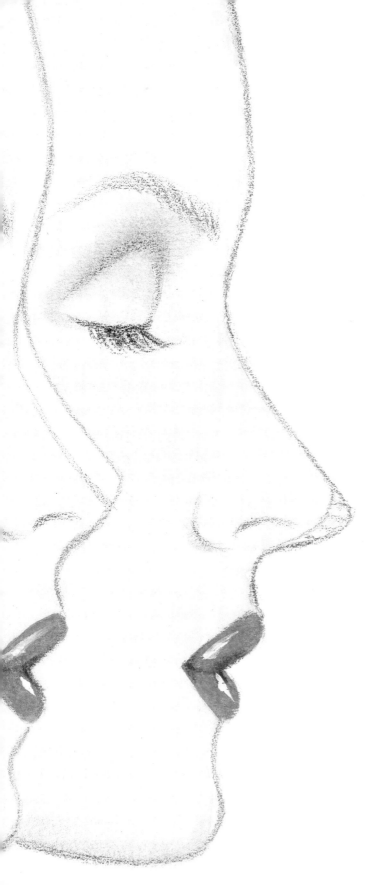

Correcting Techniques: Nose

If you want to modify the shape of your nose, you'll need to work with darker and/or lighter correcting colors. But keep them subtle. You don't want to call attention to the very characteristic you're trying to camouflage. And obvious sculpting is sure to draw attention. A base only half a tone lighter or darker than your normal shade is sufficient to suggest a new shape. If the change you want is more dramatic, you may want to consider cosmetic surgery. A good makeup, after all, is only an optical illusion, not a structural one. (You can also modify the width of your nose usually by altering the eyebrow-to-mouth relationship.) But by a subtle play of light and dark on the nose, you can counter several obvious characteristics.

Skinny and Short
Shade the bridge of the nose and highlight along the sides, including the nostrils.

Hooked
Offset a high arch by shading any areas of curvature on the bridge.

Broad and Flat
Use a lighter base on the bridge and shade the sides, including the nostrils.

Turned Up
Use a lighter base on the bridge to make it appear higher. This will match the top part to the tilt.

Long
Shadow just underneath the tip, especially if the end turns downward.

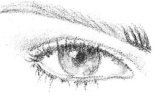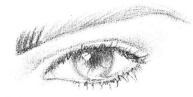

The shape of your eyebrows and mouth can affect how people perceive the width of your nose. Lining up the inside corner of your eyebrows with the base of your nose will narrow a wide nose and widen a thin one. The relationship of the top of the lips to the bottom of the nose also plays a part. Here's how it's done:

Thin Nose ▶

Make your nose seem more prominent by aligning the eyebrows with the base of the nose. Fill in the brows, matching them to the width of the base of your nose. Decrease the distance between nose and mouth by making the upper lip look thicker.

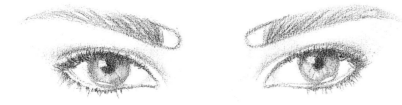

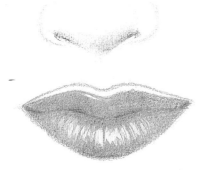

◀ Wide Nose

Tweeze the inside corners of your eyebrows to line up with the base of your nose. A wider space between your eyes will bring the focus up and away from your nose. Then elongate the line between mouth and nose by narrowing just the upper lip.

Correcting Techniques: Undereye Bags

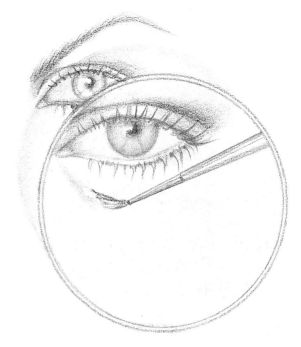

Most women look at bags, pouches, or circles under the eyes as a sign of aging. True, bags can result from a weakening of skin tone, a loss of elasticity, or a thinning of the skin texture. But they can just as easily be the result of too much sleep, too little sleep, a sinus condition, or an allergy. Whatever the reason, pouchy-looking eyes can be distressing at any age. Here are some suggestions for camouflaging undereye bags:

- Soothe your eyes by relaxing for three minutes with chamomile tea bags placed on top of each closed lid.

- Apply your foundation first. If you have pouches or puffy bags, use a base half a tone darker than your normal shade on these areas. If you have deep circles, use a base half a tone lighter.

- Apply a lighter concealer color to the blue-shadowed areas under the eye only. Use it on eyelids too if they are dark. Never put concealer on the swollen, pouchy areas.

- Apply loose powder to the undereye area with a brush. Don't press it on, as you do with the rest of your face. Set the powder under the eye area by running your little finger lightly around the rim of the eye socket. This will even out the powder, so it won't stay on top of the skin and emphasize any wrinkles.

- Pay extra attention to your lashes. A clumpy mascara application will make the whole eye area look dirty.

- Don't use mauve, pink, blue, or purple shades of eye shadow. They simply repeat the very colors you want to get rid of in the dark circles.

- Don't use black or dark-colored pencils around the eyes. On puffy days, use a light gray.

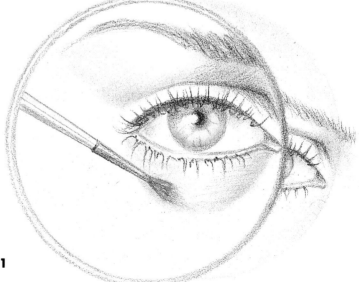

Correcting Techniques: Eyes

Your eyes are what give expression to your face. They reveal your thoughts, emotions, desires, and fears—even when you don't want them to. And they'll do this no matter what shape they are, no matter what makeup you use. So why worry about correcting their shape? Because, in addition to being your most expressive feature, your eyes give balance to your face. Their very set and shape influences the relationship among all other facial features. Where you place your blush is always in proportion to your eyes; how you balance your nose is always in direct relationship with your eyes. Even the width of your mouth should correspond to the set of your eyes. All these are reasons to give your eyes the attention they deserve.

Start by drawing a line of color just under the lower lashes. Don't stroke from side to side on the shadow pan. Instead, hold the sponge-tip applicator straight up and down, and get the color just at the tip. Take it from lighter to darker at the outside corner, feathering the color out. Then smudge the entire line to give it subtlety.

To shade the lid area, deposit the color at the outside corner and press down. This keeps the color particles from falling below the eye. Then blend color up and out over the lid going from dark to light.

Next, use a highlighting shadow to contour the curve of the eye. Add a lighter shade, depositing all color on the inside corner of your eye. Bring this highlighting up and out, overlapping the darker edge of your first shadow. Never leave a rainbow effect, with one color just meeting the edge of another; overlap the edges for a softer effect.

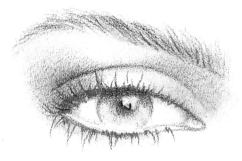
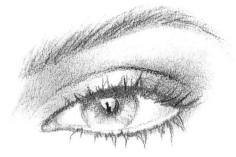

Almond Shaped ▲

Almond eyes are the ideal shape, adapting to all kinds of fashion. Accentuate the graceful curves by shadowing the inner and outermost part of the lids, extending up and out slightly. Place a bit of lighter highlight color just in the center of the lid and under the brow arch. Add color beneath the lower lashes. Apply mascara to both upper and lower lashes, extending it the full length of the eye.

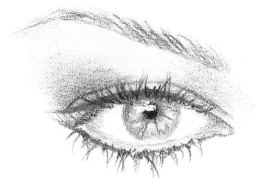
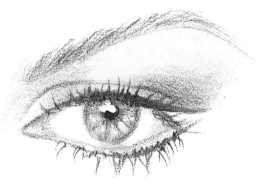

Droopy ▲

Start with eyeliner close to the lashline on the inside corner of the eye. Take it three quarters of the way across the lashline, then sweep it up beyond the natural eye corner. Use shadow in the crease, following the curve of the eyeliner. Sweep up the shadow where the eyeliner sweeps upward. Extend beyond the outside eye corner. Apply mascara only to those lashes that are before this line; leave lashes that fall after the extended line alone. With an eye pencil, parallel the eyeliner just underneath the lower lashes. Sweep it up at the outside corner at a similar slant. Do not let the two lines meet. Use mascara all the way across the lower lashes.

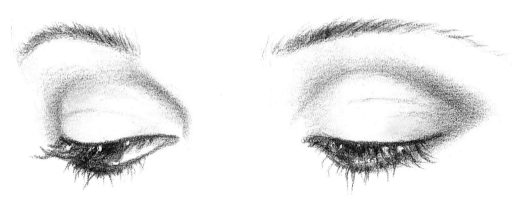

Deep Set ▲

Create the illusion of a higher natural eye crease by using a dark shadow above the crease line. Apply a lighter shadow in the crease and continue below it. Never put a dark color in the crease. Add a highlight color just above the dark shadow. Line the upper lid just at the base of the lashes, extending the line upward as the continuation of the last lash. Use lots of mascara all around the eye.

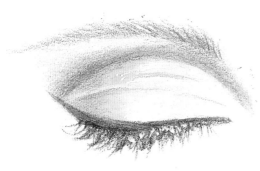
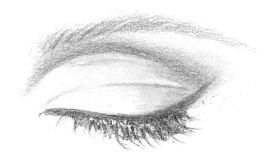

Narrow Lidded ▲

Use two deep-toned pencils and a shadow, all in the same color family, to create a crease. Begin with the lighter pencil, drawing a new crease line from the top of the lid across the eye down to the corners of the lashes. Smudge with a cotton swab. Go over the same line with shadow to blend. Use the darker pencil to draw a line along the base of the lashes, bringing it up and out at the corners to the new crease line. Continue the shadow across the lid.

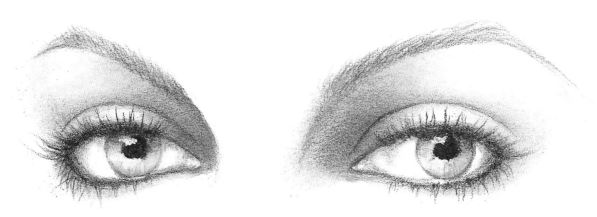

Too Far Apart ▲

Accentuate the inner corner of the eye with darker colors toward the bridge of the nose; use lighter colors at the outer corners. Apply shadow right next to the nose, then fill in the wedge from eye to brow. Reverse the mascara technique for eyes that are close set; concentrate the third and fourth layers on the inside-to-middle lashes. Bring your eyebrows closer to the nose bone.

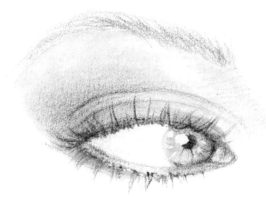 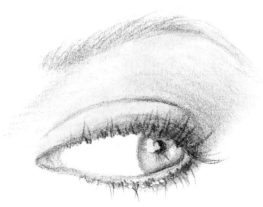

Close Set ▲

Put the accent on the outside corners of the eye. That's where the color should be the darkest, the lashes should be the longest, and the lines should be the most obvious. But don't forget to blend it—lightly—to the inner corner area. It's too obvious if the color doesn't con-tinue. The first two layers of mascara should be swept across all lashes; the last two layers should cover the outer lashes only. Create the illusion of wider-spaced eyes by carefully tweezing the eyebrows. Remove a triangle just at the nose bone.

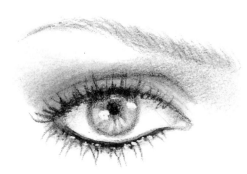 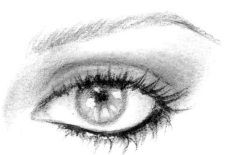

Bulging ▲

Cover the upper lid with a dark shadow (smoky gray or brown), extending it above the natural crease. Rim the lower lashes with a line just inside the eye. Make your mascara more prominent on the middle lashes, upper and lower. Use highlight shadow only under the arch. Do not sweep it across the upper brow-bone area. The trick is to make the eye recede. Add the attraction of color just beneath the lower lashes.

Correcting Techniques: Forehead and Jawline

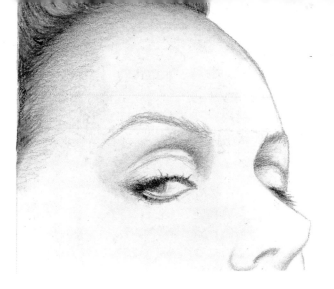

Shading along the hairline or just at the base of your face helps to minimize a high forehead, a square jaw, a double chin, or a long face. But there are ways to do it. You don't want to rub color carelessly across.

Square Jaw ▼
Avoid the natural cheek shadow of a square jaw when you begin to shade. Put the darkest color only on the most extended part of the jawline. Blend so that the roundest part is the darkest, shading lighter and lighter toward the center.

High Forehead ▲
Lessen the demarcation between skin color and hair color by shading in a darker, oval area next to the hairline. This helps to soften the brightness of a high forehead and creates a rounder shape for the face. Narrow the shading as it approaches the temples.

Long Face, Double Chin ▼
Use a darker color just under the jawline, blending from lighter at the outside to deeper in the center. (If you don't have a long face or a double chin, leave this area alone.)

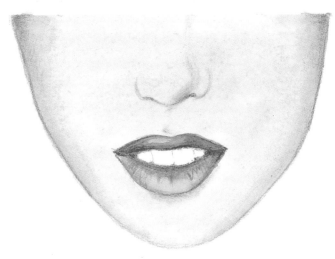

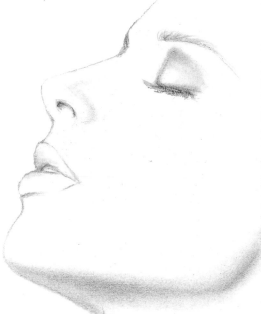

Correcting Techniques: Lips

Your lips are the second biggest attention getters on your face. They can be bright or pale, but as long as they are beautifully finished with color they give a focus to the face. And they make your eye makeup seem that much more important.

To find the perfect lip proportion for your face, draw an imaginary line from the inner rim of the iris of your eye (when staring straight ahead) down to the corners of your mouth. This is the ideal width for your lips. No lip liner or color should extend beyond this point.

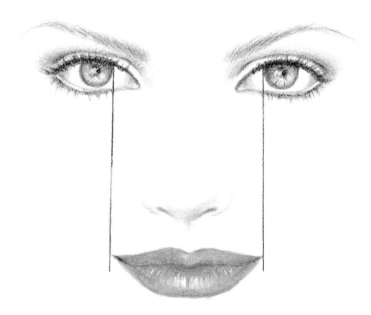

If you start by outlining your lips with pencil, your lip color will stay within the boundaries with less likelihood of "bleeding" into the lines around your mouth. And your lip shape will be prettily defined. Nothing makes as much difference as this. When selecting your lip pencil shade, go only about half a tone darker than your normal lipstick color. The brown line that some women think looks more natural only tends to make the mouth recede.

Start with the pencil in the middle of your lower lip and line outward to the corners. Repeat the same center-to-corner technique on top. For lip color that lasts longer than even the longest-lasting lipstick, fill in lips with the pencil. Powder, then put your lipstick over.

Always use a lipstick brush to apply lipstick, but do not put the brush directly to the tube. Instead, scrape a small amount of lipstick off with a tiny plastic spatula. This softens the lipstick into a butterlike consistency and makes it much easier to apply. Dip the brush into it, really roll it around, and coat the tip with color. To apply, start with the brush smack in the center of your lower lip and spread the color out evenly from there. Do not begin at the corners of your lips, or you'll glob all the color at the narrowest spot. Follow these techniques:

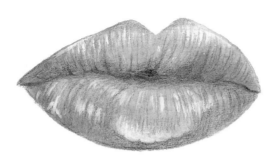

◄ Crinkly Lips

Use lots of shine to draw attention away from the crinkles. A matte finish only makes lines more obvious. Just apply color and gloss. Don't outline lips with a darker pencil; don't powder. Just remember, the more your lips shine, the less your crinkles will show. Use petroleum jelly at bedtime to soften lips through the night.

Thick Lips ►

Cover your lips with base. Use a pencil half a shade darker than your lipstick to draw your ideal lip shape just inside your natural lip line. Powder over to soften the line. Fill in your new lip shape with lipstick.

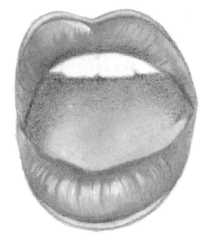

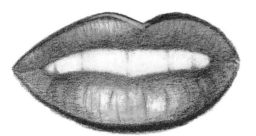

◄ Thin Lips

Apply base over your lips. Then outline the shape you want above your natural lip line with a pencil in a shade darker than your principal lipstick color. Next, use a small, thin brush to apply a shade of lipstick in the same color family as the pencil to the area between the pencil line and the natural lip line. Powder over. Finally, apply your principal lipstick color, up to and covering the original darker pencil line.

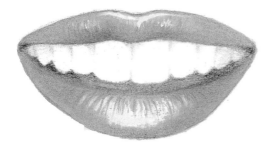

◄ Flat Lips

Add curvature by filling in lips with color, except at the center. Use a lighter, iridescent shade at the center or add a spot of gloss. Don't powder. It's the shine that gives the shape.

Puckered Lips ►

Smooth out the tiny vertical lines around the mouth by stretching your lips between the second and third fingers so that lip color goes on evenly. First, outline lips with a dry pencil. The less greasy the color is just at the ridge of the lip line, the less it will bleed into the tiny lines. Powder over pencil and fill in with lipstick, just to the inside rim of the pencil line.

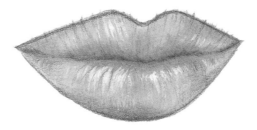

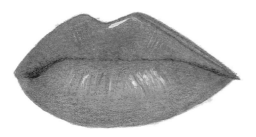

◄ Uneven Lips

Cover lips with base. Balance any uneven part by outlining the desired shape with a darker lip pencil. Fill in the area between the pencil line and the natural lip line with a dark lipstick in the same range as the lip pencil. Powder, then apply a lighter lipstick shade to the entire mouth, up to and covering the drawn line.

Droopy Lips ►

Cover the natural lip line at corners with a concealer stick. Blend well. Lift the outer corners with a pencil line. Begin by extending the lower lip, taking the line upward. It should touch and go just a bit above the upper lip corner. Then extend the upper lip line to meet it. Set and soften the pencil line with powder and fill in with color.

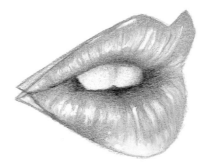

Step by Step to a Perfect Makeup

Most of this chapter has been devoted to techniques for enhancing the form of your face and its features. But to achieve a harmonious overall effect, these techniques must be integrated into a basic makeup routine you can use *all* the time.

A five-minutes-in-the-morning beauty routine simply does not allow enough time to do a complete makeup. On the other hand, you don't want to spend an hour on your face either. Unless you're preparing a very elaborate, fantasy makeup, anything more than twenty minutes is a waste of time. (If you want to upgrade your makeup throughout the day, see pages 86–89 for a morning-into-evening makeup strategy.) With more time, you may be tempted to do more, and an overdone face is just as inappropriate as an underdone one.

I do not count your cleansing/toning/moisturizing time in these twenty minutes. You must bring to the task a properly prepared "canvas"—and begin from there. Your makeup will go on much more smoothly, the colors will remain true for a longer time, and the skin will respond with more suppleness if your face has been properly treated before applying cosmetics.

The Proper Position

Before you begin your makeup, learn how to get the most from your mirror. It is always best to sit at a table facing a mirror, rather than stand in front of one. A table gives you something to lean your elbows on, which automatically steadies your hand. If you must stand, use your opposite hand to cup the elbow of the arm you are using. This will stabilize the arm and keep your hand from getting the jitters. Begin with the side of the face that is opposite to your natural hand. For instance, a right-handed person should start with the left side of her face. This will be the more difficult side to do, and it will be easier to match the right side to the left side than vice versa.

The best way to apply eye makeup is to position the mirror under the chin. Look down at it, keeping your head straight (don't bend your neck downward). You should be able to see the entire surface of your eyelid without pulling the skin or wrinkling the lid. By applying your eye makeup with a downward glance at a mirror, you'll be sure to use color effectively on the *entire* lid. It's a big mistake to cover only the portion of the lid you can see with your eyes *open*.

A perfectly made-up face is the result of selecting the right colors and putting them in the right places! But no matter which shades and shading techniques you choose, there is a basic procedure to follow when you want to put makeup on so that it stays on. You can't skip steps if you want the effect to last. And remember, makeup is much more effective when it is built up slowly, with lots of light little layers. Never settle for one product that claims to do everything (a base and a powder combined, for instance). If you get heavy-handed with any single product in order to save time, it will be obvious. Makeup becomes much more beautiful and transparent when it is applied in subtle layers.

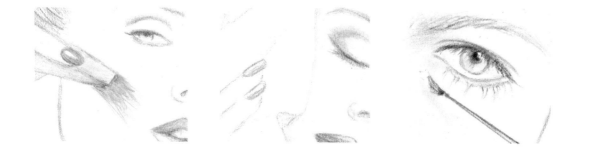

1. Start

Begin with absolutely clean skin. Makeup won't stay on skin that hasn't been properly cleansed.

2. Moisturize and Blot

Apply moisturizer to your entire face. Poke a hole for your nose through the center of a facial tissue, put the tissue over your entire face, and press lightly. You must absorb any remnants of excess moisturizer, or your makeup will move right off your face!

3. Apply Base and Blot

This is not a step to rush. A badly applied base makes the skin look shiny and the complexion look artificial. Anything indiscreet will ruin the rest of your makeup. After your base is applied, don't forget to blot. Use the same tissue technique you used for blotting your moisturizer.

4. Hold It

If you want your makeup to last all day, wait three minutes before you put another thing on your face. Use this time to file your nails, put your rollers in, take your rollers out—anything as long as you aren't tempted to touch your face.

5. Hide It

Use a thin brush to place a light-colored concealer just under the eye area. Position it *only* where you see a blue shadow. Finish by adding a dot of concealer on the outside corner of the eye.

6. Highlight It

Continue using your concealer to highlight the planes of your face. Put a dot in the center of your forehead; a stroke down the center of your nose; two commas on the sides of your nostrils; two apostrophes at the corners of your mouth; a final dot at the center of the chin. Think of it as face punctuation. And blend everything!

7. Powder and Press

Whether you like a matte finish or not, powder is what makes your makeup stay put. It is a myth that powder accentuates wrinkles. It can, but only if improperly applied. You never want powder to sit on top of your makeup. When your body heat warms the base, it will start to move—and so will the powder on top of it—right into every crevice!

You must make your powder *one* with the base. Make sure you use only loose powder at this point. Compacts are for retouching.

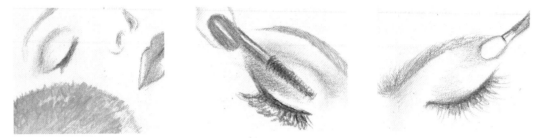

Don't dust the first application of powder on with a brush. Think, instead, of fusing the powder into the base. Take a big square of dry cotton, fold the edges in, and use a rolling motion to press/release, press/release the powder over your face, eyelids, and lips. If you press powder into your face this way, it will always be transparent no matter how much you use.

If you prefer a "dewy," unpowdered effect, you can bring back the glow by wetting a cotton ball with a mild astringent. Press the cotton against your face (everywhere except the nose area). This will take away the powdered look without removing anything. The alcohol in the astringent will also "fix" the makeup immediately. I recommend this trick especially for evening makeup.

If you do like a matte look but wish to fix your makeup with astringent, simply repowder lightly, after blotting, with a powder brush.

In the summer, pay particular attention to powdering the T-zone area. A shiny forehead and nose do not make any woman more attractive!

8. Build Mascara

Start applying your mascara with a single stroke of the wand on each eye. You'll eventually want four thin layers on your lashes. If you start now, allowing time for each layer to dry and to comb lashes in between, you'll avoid the thick, clumpy, overmascara'd look that results from trying to add too many coats at the last minute. An early stroke of mascara begins to give a certain shape to the eye, a balance to the face. You need this definition *before* you begin to apply eye makeup.

9. Add Eye Shadow

After your eyes are framed with their first layer of mascara, you'll have a better sense of the form of the eye to follow in applying shadow.

Use the shadow-shaping technique that best suits the shape of your eyes. Line the lower lashes first, then stroke on your lid color. Apply another coat of mascara, then add your highlighting shade on the browbone. Finish with another coat of mascara.

10. Begin to Blush

It would be helpful if you could make your face blush naturally to see where the color comes to your cheeks; then you could apply your favorite shade to the spot. But even if you can't, remember that blusher should look as natural as a blush. Use a long-handled brush to keep your hand light.

(See pages 48–55 for blusher face-shaping techniques.)

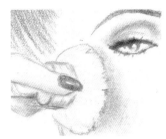 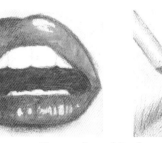 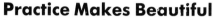

A little blusher on the outside corners of your browbone will tone down any obvious shadow colors and blend the eye makeup in.

11. Emphasize the Eyebrows

Use a combination of two pencil colors. And take your time—this can't be rushed. (For perfect brow shaping, see page 56.) Add more mascara.

12. Color Lips

To make the color last longer, always apply two layers. Blot the first with a tissue, then reapply. (For correct lip measurements, see page 67.)

13. Pat on Powder

A final touch of powder from a compact will smooth the finished effect. Lightly press the formulated powder into the sides and bridge of the nose, the forehead, the temples, and the chin.

14. Check the Mirror

No makeup is ever complete without one last look. Before you go out, always verify—by daylight, if possible—that your final makeup is not too vivid, that everything is well blended.

Practice Makes Beautiful

Now that you know the techniques and tricks of applying makeup, you've got to put in some practice time. And not five minutes before you have to go out! Never experiment when you haven't the time to take everything off and try again. Save it for Sunday. You need time, daylight, and an easygoing attitude that will allow you to exaggerate everything. It's always best to overdo every line, every color, every shading when you're trying something new. It should be shocking or it isn't worth doing. When you make a mistake, make a big one. You can always tone it down. If you don't apply color heavily enough at first, or if you blend it too much, you won't see the effect you're trying to create at all.

Once you like what you see in the mirror, check it by daylight. Tone it down, if necessary. Look again. If you're satisfied with the results, write down everything you did, every color you used—and tape your notes to your mirror. Don't think you'll remember the next time. Practice the same technique over and over until you're confident and until you can do the whole job in less than twenty minutes. Experiment within different color palettes and practice coordinating new harmonies of color. You'll soon have the basis of a beauty routine that will last through the looks of a lifetime.

Anouk Aimée: Her very feminine look and expressive, perfectly shaped face call for muted tones, wines, and smokes; lots of bright color would overpower her delicate features.

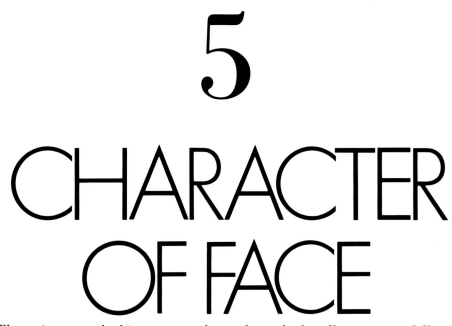

5
CHARACTER OF FACE

There is no such thing as a makeup formula for all women to follow.
No one wants to look just like someone else.

Every woman has physical characteristics that require special makeup considerations. Corrective techniques for certain features were covered in the Form of Face chapter. Other characteristics do not require change as much as they do an acknowledgment of their existence and an awareness of techniques that will incorporate them into a personal beauty style. For example, a black woman needs to factor special tone and structure considerations into makeup application. Asiatic women must emphasize eyes differently, select colors differently. A woman with white hair must learn how to co-exist with it. And women with eyeglasses must learn how to incorporate them into an unobtrusive beauty look. It is wrong to assume that a single makeup technique applies to women of every age. Yet people often do, failing to take into account the fact that makeup and skin needs change as a woman ages. It is a continual process of evolution. And there is no reason why it cannot be a beautiful one.

The good news is, you can personalize your makeup to your heritage, your age, your lifestyle, your features, your individualistic traits. And all these special situations will be covered in this chapter.

Fashion and Makeup

In every season, year in and year out, there is fashion news. A new color, a new shape, a new feeling sweeps through the fashion press, the media, the runways, and ultimately the stores. It is a worldwide phenomenon, from the elegant couture salons in Europe to the chic designer houses in America. Trends begin to take shape, to grab hold, and sooner or later the best of the new fashions find their way into your closet.

Whether you have a weakness for every new thing you see or stick to one style of dressing, you will be affected by at least two important elements of fashion change: *color* and *mood*. Just as there is a new palette (and usually a dominant new color) every season, so there is also a specific mood shift that accompanies it. Severe man-tailored looks may set the tone; or romantic, feminine, nostalgic looks; or slick, sophisticated styles. Whatever the look, the new fashion colors and mood will play a key role in how you plan your makeup.

Makeup, like clothes, must reflect a sense of staying current. If it does not, things will begin to go wrong with the way your total look adds up. Something will seem to be out of focus, out of place. Makeup and fashion must mesh. When miniskirts and Mary Quant innocence became popular in the 1960s, the face had to get stronger to offset the childlike effect. So the eyes became bolder, more exaggerated. Lashes were drawn on, glued on, added on. No color was subtle, no line was blended. With the eyes so obvious, a bright mouth would have been too much. That's when white-lightened lipstick came to the rescue. A change in makeup was brought on by the change in fashion.

When makeup doesn't change to accommodate a new fashion mood, the fashion doesn't work—and it is quickly discarded. The maxiskirts of the early 1970s called for a softening of makeup colors to respond to the duller rusts, burgundies, and smoky, dusty tones of this new fashion look. But most women still held on to their "mini" faces, with op-art eyes and pale little mouths. The look didn't work because the face didn't change. Today skirts are often as long as or longer than they were in the era of the maxi. But they don't shock because the face that's worn with them has become softer, more natural.

After the awkwardness of the maxi, we had the age of commonality. Anything that suggested class distinction was discarded. Jewelry and elegance lost out to jeans and T-shirts. Everyone wanted to be tan and shiny and natural and young. That's when clear, transparent makeup came in: gels, glosses, bronzers. Everything took on a brown tone, even lips. Coral, beige, and brown lip colors replaced anything with pink in it. And eye makeup toned way down.

Things didn't brighten up again until hats made a comeback in the early 1980s. When a brim casts a shadow from your forehead to your nose, your lips and cheeks had better stand out. There must be a focus somewhere on the face. So colors once again began to go darker, get brighter.

Fashion continues to grow more sophisticated. There is a body consciousness, a movement to clothes now. Nothing is stiff and artificial, especially around the face. Hair must move and be upkeep-free. Makeup must not look like it took two hours to apply—but it must be there. The scrubbed and healthy look is no longer enough. Clothes are becoming stronger.

You need a certain amount of makeup today, a certain sophistication, if you are wearing the bolder colors, the bigger looks. Whatever you do, your eyes must be there; your mouth must be there. But this time, you're not hardening your face and you're not hiding it. You are simply affirming its existence in a very natural, uncontrived way.

The "New" You

Accommodating fashion shifts into your overall look doesn't mean you have to change. In fact, if you do change drastically, you won't be comfortable with yourself—and it will show. It's easy to feel silly when you wear something that you never should have bought in the first place. So the first rule for selecting the correct fashion face for you is: *Be very comfortable in what you choose to wear.* You can incorporate new fashion trends into your wardrobe without letting them take over entirely. A brighter blazer might be your token nod to a season of electric colors. You might signal the romantic in you by a simple lace handkerchief or tailored white linen blouse, without resorting to ruffles and flourishes. Or a tailored, tweedy coat might be as close as you'll ever want to get to the haberdashery look. The point is to be true to your own fashion style. Know the kind of person you *really* are. Sophisticated? Sporty? Experimental? Then plan your fashion selection—and your makeup—around your favorite way of being. Your makeup will always look right if you have the right attitude to go with the clothes.

This does not mean that you should stay with the same old face! Just as you add new fashion touches to your wardrobe, so you must find the appropriate makeup touches for each fashion look.

With a natural makeup, the emphasis is on creating true skin tones, true color placement. With a sophisticated makeup, you can concentrate more on coverage and on color. It's never the *amount* of makeup that determines the effect. The legendary Hollywood beauties of the 1930s and 1940s created very sophisticated looks by focusing only on eyebrows, lashes, and lips. And they certainly didn't have the variety of colors and products that we have today.

The Three Faces of Fashion

The names for the new fashion trends change each season. One year we have gypsies, the next year Yugoslavian peasants, the next year Moroccan nomads. But the message is always the same: *exotic.* Or we go from Victorian heroine to Proustian ingenue, and the mood is always *romantic.* What goes with polo ponies one year and fox hunts the next is always sedately *sporty.* And anything from Newport to Deauville calls up instant images of refined *elegance.* No matter how the fashion translations change year in and year out, these basic fashion types remain constant. And we must always keep one category open for the *trendy:* anything shocking, new, innovative. What's startling may change each time around, but the fact that fashion *can* shock does not.

You can find your fashion type easily with a quick glance at your closet. The clothes you already own will give you a clear indication of the fashion looks you feel most comfortable in. Unless you're incredibly disciplined, all your clothes won't reflect the same fashion mood, but a majority of them will be exotic, romantic, sporty, elegant, or trendy.

If you are a true romantic, for instance, you may be wearing French schoolgirl looks one season and long white linen skirts the

---

SEASONAL FACES

The makeup strategy described below has nothing to do with color "types" described in other books. Rather, it is a seasonal guide to wearing the right makeup at the right time.

The Spring Face
Take the first spring days to investigate the new shades just starting to appear in the stores. Think light, clean colors. Your first purchase: a brighter blush to add warmth to your skin.

The Summer Face
If you like to play with colors, don't get too tan. The contrast is too alarming. Play up the eyes, go easier on the lips. Lighten up makeup with sheer colors, translucent formulations. Now is the time to let your natural glow show.

The Fall Face
The new fall shades are introduced by early September. Begin to experiment with colors that *don't* go with a tan. Your palette can be richer, deeper, more dramatic.

The Winter Face
Warm up your color palette. A pale mouth in winter just looks cold! Emphasize lips and cheeks with colors that warm up the face. Try a sheer bronzing gel over your moisturizer for days when you just have to have a tan.

next. You'll adjust for the colors of the new season, but your makeup will stay true to your style: softly romantic. The best makeup approach for this look is *natural*. Similarly, if you live in tweeds and shetlands in the winter and wear only natural fabrics in the summer, you're at your best in a relaxed, sporty clothes. The best makeup strategy for you, too, is natural.

An elegant, polished wardrobe demands a *sophisticated* makeup. Your clothes will have impact; your face must too. And if you favor tailored executive looks, sophisticated makeup will suit as well.

Any look from exotic to trendy needs a more *colorful* makeup approach. If you're at all experimental in your fashion looks, you must create an equally interesting face. Anything too soft, too subtle, will pale by comparison.

These three basic makeup strategies—natural, sophisticated, and colorful—are detailed for you in this chapter. Your main objective will be to find the face that goes with your predominant fashion style. But you will also learn the tricks that turn a face from natural to sophisticated, from sophisticated to colorful, so that no matter what you are wearing you can always adapt your face to your fashion.

No one represents the face of contemporary fashion more than Brooke Shields. A naturally beautiful young woman whose face has adorned the covers of magazines across the world, she represents a truly international standard of beauty.

Her beauty may not be your beauty, but there is a lesson to be learned in the adaptability of her face—of her attitude—to every fashion look. Photographers remark that she does not simply wear clothes; she *becomes* them. That must happen when you are creating an appearance to project a specific fashion mood. It's all in the attitude. If you don't feel like the woman you're made up to be, nobody else will believe you are either. And no makeup tricks will turn you into something you're not.

If you can carry off a personality switch, all three of the following fashion faces may be right for you at one time or another. If you prefer to stick to a certain style, choose the face that best matches your wardrobe preference.

THE NATURAL FACE

Natural never means naked. The moment you begin to enhance your appearance with one beauty product, you've got to go through with the whole thing. You don't get results by making up just a part of your face. To women who say, "I only use a little mascara" or "I only do my eyes," I say, why bother? You're only throwing something out of balance. And that's the farthest thing from a natural look. Our eyes go immediately to the one part of the face that's been dramatized.

To look naturally beautiful means having no distractions of color on the face. A truly natural makeup is neutral enough to go with everything. Concentrate on creating true skin tones that blend with the tones you already have.

1. Apply Base and Blot

Select a light base (a cream gel is less covering than any other kind of base) if your skin is in good condition. The amount of coverage will depend on your complexion; but for a natural finish it should always be on the light side.

2. Cover and Highlight

Use a concealer, and cover with a very translucent powder applied with a brush.

3. Build Mascara

Add subtle eye emphasis with smudged pencil (black, brown, or gray) around the eye, then apply two or three layers of mascara. Comb lashes carefully between coats; clumping looks anything but natural.

4. Add Blush

The only cheek color to add is a natural-looking earth powder. In a reddish-brown tone, it will warm up the complexion like the sun, without looking like a specific blush color. Add a bit to your eyelids for natural emphasis.

5. Color Lips

Match lip color to the basic tone of your lips. You could go a half shade darker or lighter, but that's it. Use a transparent gloss. Apply it with fingers, then blot half of it away. Or use your earth blush on your lips. Apply with fingertip, top with gloss, and blot.

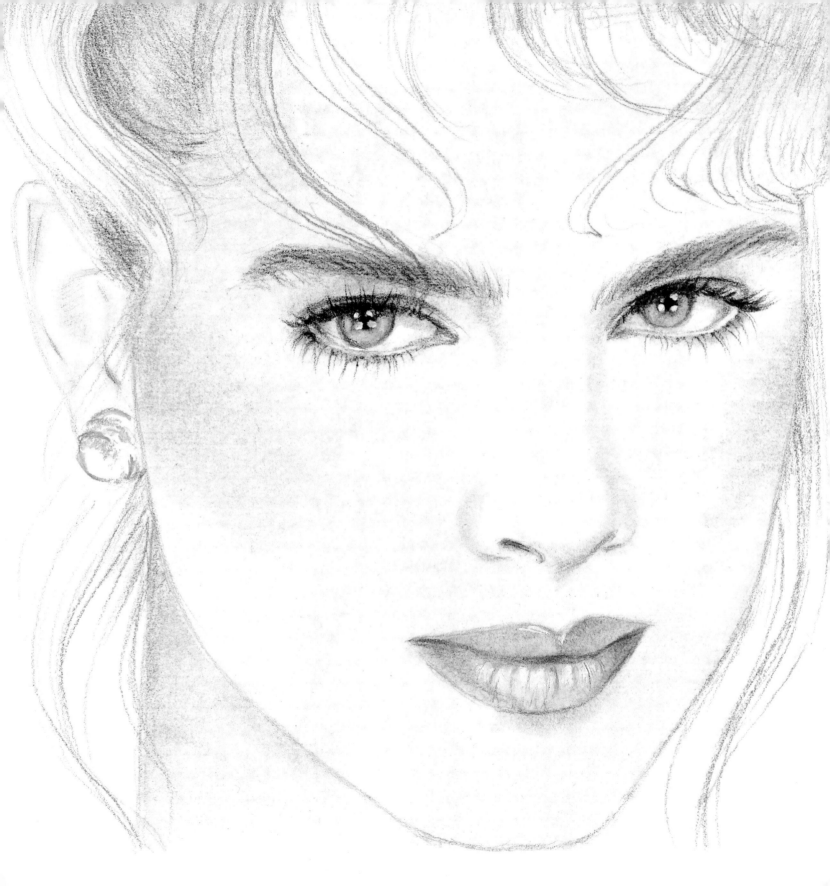

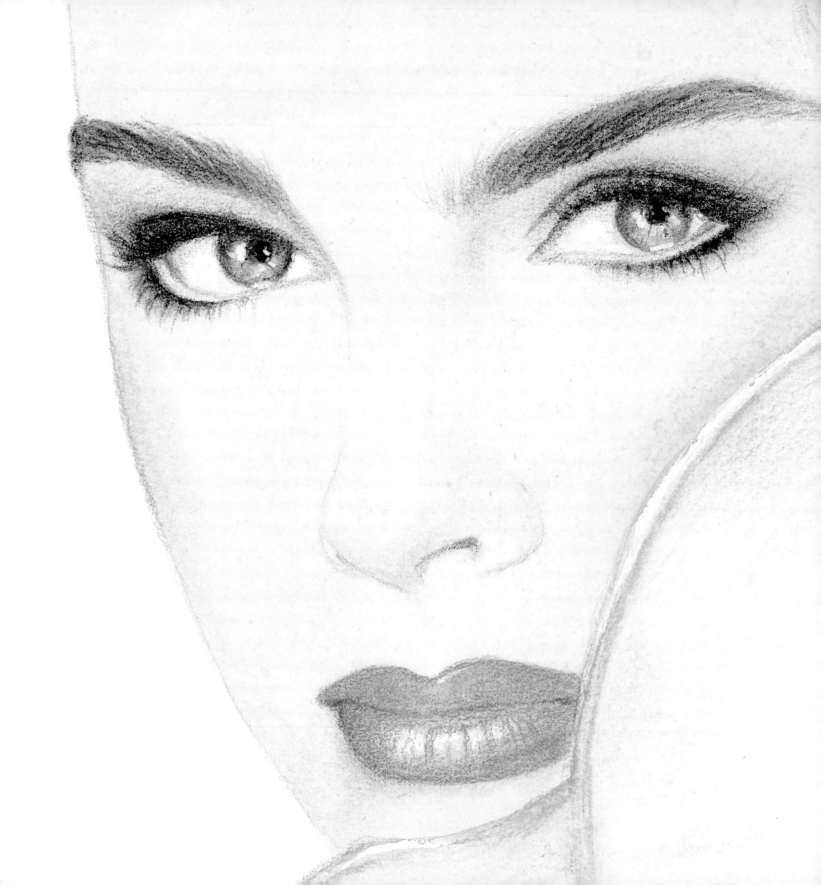

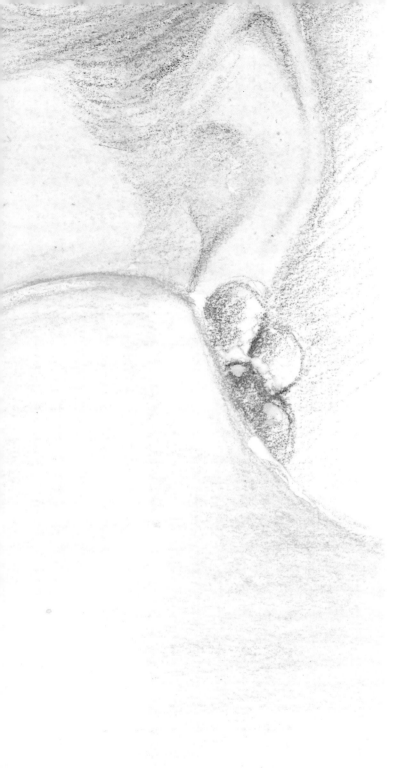

THE SOPHISTICATED FACE

The more makeup coverage you have, the more sophisticated your look becomes. You can create a perfect matte effect with a very thin film of makeup. Sophisticated doesn't mean thick. It means nontransparent.

1. Apply Base and Blot

Start with a cream base, applied evenly and lightly.

2. Cover and Highlight

Blend away shadows with concealer, then top with a nontranslucent powder. Press in for a soft matte finish.

3. Add Blush

Use a soft powder blush. (Cream blushes add shine, and shine is not sophisticated.)

4. Emphasize Eyes

Play up your eyes—make them smoky, mysterious. Use powder shadow on the lids, combined with pencils to rim the eyes. For a more exotic touch, pencil a thin rim *inside*. (Since an inner rim tends to make the eyes smaller, this is not a technique for anyone with narrow eyes.) Add lots of mascara, using a colored mascara for the last layers.

5. Color Lips

Use muted and matte lip color—no startling brights, no sparkling frosts. Stay with stronger shades.

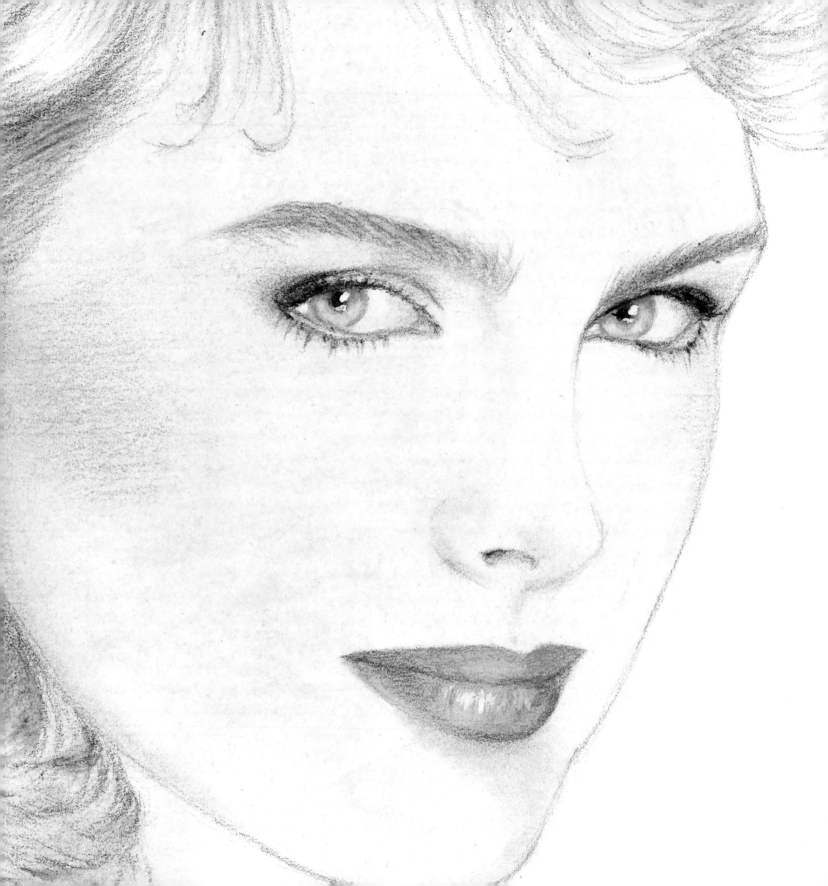

THE COLORFUL FACE

Certain clothes call for a colorful makeup. Without it, your face will lose its importance. But you must never compete color for color. It's impact you're after. If too much is going on with what you're wearing, a colorful makeup will be too much. The colorful face is at its best with clothes that make a strong single-color statement.

The predominating color in what you're wearing will determine the color play of your makeup. But don't get stuck in a one-color rut. Use a contrasting color to break it up—on your lashes, under your eyes, on your lips. Apply a gold-tinged blusher, add a blue line under the eyes, and top your lashes with blue mascara. Use some restraint, of course. When you're playing with strong tones, one or two contrasting shades is quite enough. With a wild print, tone your face down to a one-color statement.

1. Apply Base and Blot
Use a neutral base to balance a colorful face. Don't start adding obvious rose tones or yellow tones, except to correct your skin's undertone. The base can be more covering than one you would use for a natural makeup, but it should not be as matte as a sophisticated makeup base. Keep it transparent and light. A fluid applied with a damp sponge or a wet-then-pressed cotton ball is best. Apply a translucent powder with a press/release motion.

2. Add Blush
Apply a blusher in the correct harmony-of-color scheme to match what you are wearing. (See Chapter 3.)

3. Color Lips
They can go lighter to balance a brighter face; they can play with color here as well. Try a two-tone effect: Use a neutral brown/orange on the outside corners of the lips, a bright pink down the middle.

4. Emphasize Eyes
Eyes for a colorful face can range from pastel to vibrant, as long as the harmony of color corresponds to your overall makeup palette. Now is the time to try a two-tone (or more!) eye shadow strategy. Play with blue/yellow, green/blue, and apricot/navy combinations. Line the eye in the same color as the mascara you select (and your mascara *can* be a color other than brown or black). Eye makeup for a colorful face should not be as dramatic as it is for a sophisticated one, but it can be slightly experimental.

When you are selecting shades for a colorful face, never judge the color by the way it looks in the pan. What you see is concentrated color. The effect you get when you stroke it on your skin is far lighter and far more natural-looking. Don't be afraid to try the wildest-looking shades at the counter. The result may be something surprisingly pretty on you.

A Round-the-Clock Makeup Strategy

If you simply cannot devote twenty minutes to your basic makeup in the morning, do *not* try to fit everything into the limited amount of time you do have. You'll only end up with a half-finished face! Instead, plan a progressive makeup strategy, one that gets you looking better as the day goes on. (After all, how much makeup do you really need for a 9:00 A.M. meeting?) If you follow the simple round-the-clock techniques outlined below, you'll always be wearing the right face at the right time—and it will take you no time at all!

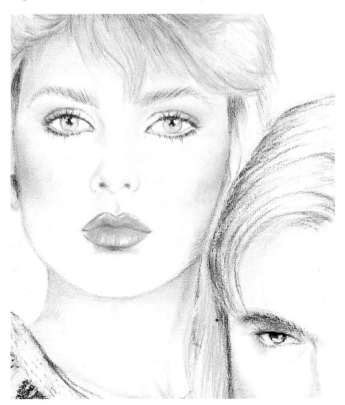

8:00 A.M.— ONLY THE BASICS

Because daylight doesn't drain red tones from your face, as artificial light does, you can get away with less makeup in the morning. Concentrate on proper cleansing, toning, and moisturizing. Here's all you'll need to do to get you out the door:

1. Apply Base and Blot
Apply either a tinted moisturizer or a moisturizing base in place of both products. This light coverage is all you'll need.

2. Powder and Press
Moisturizing powder adds an extra layer of moisture protection.

3. Blush a Bit
A dusting of blush is plenty for this time of day, and can be intensified as the day wears on.

4. Add a Little Lash
One layer will suffice and look more natural with this minimal makeup.

5. Finish Lips
Add a sweep of lipstick or, if you prefer, a sheer or tinted lip gloss.

Take more time on your hair than on your makeup. A woman can walk out on the street with light makeup and shining, well-shaped hair and look wonderful. But if she has perfect makeup and messy hair, she'll look unfinished.

12:00 P.M.—
WORK ON THE EYES

When you start with only a very basic makeup in the morning, you'll need to tote a supply of cosmetics with you to develop your look throughout the day. To save space in your bag, look for a small, all-in-one compact that contains interchangeable eye, lip, and face colors. Or keep a spare mini makeup kit, stocked with the items suggested in Chapter 1 ("The Minimum Makeup to Take"), in your desk.

The light at midday becomes right for more eye makeup. Simply take five minutes before you leave for lunch for these few steps:

1. Add More Mascara
Apply a second layer of mascara; let dry and comb.

2. Highlight the Eyes
Add a sweep of shadow on the outside of the lid; a stroke of neutral highlighter from the center of the lid to the browbone.

3. Add Definition
A rim of darker eye pencil, applied just at the lower lash base and smudged, puts new focus on the eyes.

4. Emphasize Brows
If needed, define and dramatize the brows a bit with at least two different eyebrow pencil shades.

5. Add More Dash to Your Lashes
Apply a third layer of mascara; let dry and comb.

6. Balance with Blush
Blusher should be reapplied, a little stronger than before, to stand up to the new intensity of your makeup.

7. Redefine Lips
As a finishing touch, refresh your lipstick, and you're off.

5:00 P.M.—
UPGRADE FOR EVENING

Night lights can fade your face, and artificial lighting can take every bit of red out. You'll have to intensify your color scheme, taking care to use red-based blusher and lip colors. Choose a pale base (the better for you to glow against). When you add sexy touches of vibrant color to your eyes and mouth, that's all you'll need.

Here are the steps to take you from daytime pretty to nighttime exciting:

1. Clean Up Your Act
Remove all traces of blusher and powder from your skin with a cleanser-soaked cotton pad. (Don't touch your eyes, or you'll have to start from scratch!)

2. Remoisturize
Pay special attention to the undereye area, cheeks, and laugh lines. Blot.

3. Apply Base and Blot
Use a water-based liquid makeup for a less dewy, more sophisticated effect.

4. Add Highlights
Use a concealer stick on the forehead, nose, mouth corners, and chin (as in Step by Step to a Perfect Makeup, step 6). Blend.

5. Powder and Press
Powder and press with cotton dampened with astringent. Repowder for a matte finish.

6. Brighten Up
Brighten your blush color for night. Go from pink to red, apricot to bronze, burgundy to plum. Blush from temple to cheekbones. Blush again at the chin.

7. Intensify Eyes
Add glow to your eye color with metallic highlight shadows. Go deeper with smoky tones in shadows and lining pencils. Extend the undereye line slightly and smudge upward, blending into a shadow of color just above.

8. Don't Ignore Your Brows
Extend your eyebrow line to equal the extended shadow area. Don't let your brows fall short. They're part of the overall proportion.

9. Get a Glow
Add a dot of blusher just at the browbone and blend.

10. Add More Mascara
Stroke on one last layer of mascara. Let dry and comb. (If you like, you can use a layer of colored mascara over your basic black or brown mascara layers.)

11. Focus on Lips
Outline the lips and fill in with pencil color. Top with lipstick (bright red is sexiest at night), and blot. Add the glow of gloss to the center of your lower lip only. Now smile!

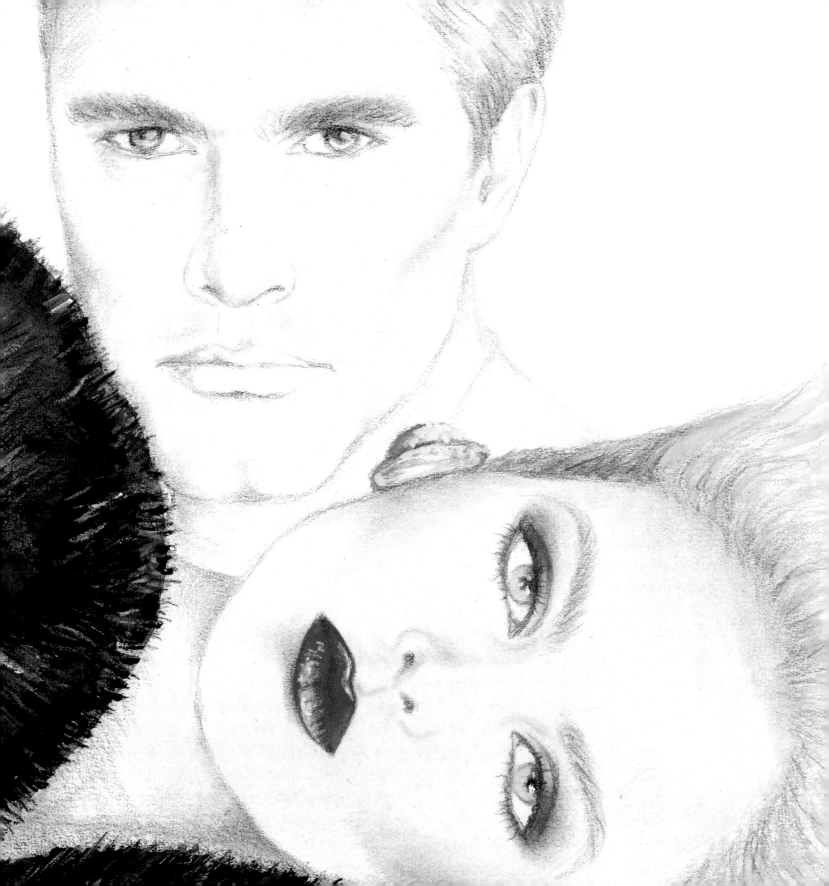

Beauty for Every Age

Too many women add more and more artificiality to their makeup as they age —when just the opposite approach is advisable. Once a woman reaches her prime, she should reveal more of herself, hide less. A woman who stays with a makeup style from younger years, either out of habit or out of fear, begins to look like a caricature of her former self. We can see on her face the exact date when she felt the most confidence in her beauty.

Ideally, as a woman becomes more confident with who she is, she should be more comfortable with her unique beauty attributes. And the makeup she selects to wear (or not to wear) should reflect this confidence.

This chapter will detail an appropriate makeup and treatment game plan for four very different stages in a woman's life. Keep in mind, however, that it is difficult to define any woman by her age. A woman of forty can have more freshness in her face, more vitality, than someone much younger in age. For such a woman, I would never suggest hiding that glow behind a sophisticated matte makeup. That's when she'll start to look her age.

Faces of very strong character don't seem to change much with the passing years, either. Of course they *do* change; the skin alters its consistency in the natural aging process. Yet we don't seem to notice. That's because the essential character of the face has taken our attention. These faces do not need a lot of makeup to be beautiful at any age.

But the fact of the matter is, we all change. Women change more than men because of the repeated monthly shifts in the skin's acidity. Complexion problems resulting from hormonal changes gradually take their toll. Sun and environmental damage also leave their traces on the face. And so does the inevitable process of aging. Through time, the quality of the skin changes. Skin cells lose water and no longer retain their firm, young plumpness. With age, the cell renewal process slows down. The skin begins to lose its elasticity as the epidermis thins. Supporting tissues under the skin start to sag, and dreaded lines and wrinkles appear.

It doesn't happen overnight. Your skin is changing all the time, and you must reevaluate its needs and monitor its signals constantly. You can't put your treatment regimen—or your makeup routine—on automatic pilot and expect to arrive at sixty-five perfectly intact. You can never make up for lost time if you wait until the signs of change become obvious.

The best strategy is to maintain your beauty throughout your lifetime. Give your skin what it needs; avoid what it doesn't. Drink lots of water (it's the best beauty tonic there is!) and get enough exercise and enough sleep. Have healthy eating and elimination habits. Avoid too much alcohol and too much salt. Stimulate your skin so that it can rejuvenate itself, and don't suffocate it under too many creams. Lasting beauty comes from *within*. No preparation in the world is going to save your face if your skin care program hasn't followed a planned, thoughtful progression throughout your lifetime.

At any age, your beauty is truly what you make it. And the face you present to the world through makeup is a reflection of the way you perceive yourself.

The four ages of beauty described in this chapter are not a strict guide to what's appropriate for your chronological age. Consult the beauty calendar within. How young do you feel? How young do you look? How young do you act? How well does your skin respond? Once you have established your own beauty age, you'll be able to find a treatment and makeup regimen that's right for you. Your only goal should be to look beautiful. And that is not necessarily the same as looking young.

NEW AWAKENINGS: 15–25

The greatest beauty asset of a very young face is the skin. True, there can be problems with overoiliness in puberty, but once it is corrected, no makeup on earth can match a youthful, glowing complexion.

At this age it is important to take care of any skin problems you have immediately, and adjust your selection of makeup products accordingly. Naturally, an aggressive acne condition requires a regimen of special care, under the direction of a dermatologist. For occasional imbalances, however, the cleansing routines for oily skin outlined in Chapter 2 should be sufficient.

This is the time to show off your skin, not conceal it behind layers of artificial color. Heavy makeup won't do anything for you but detract from your own natural beauty. Women spend millions every year trying to recapture the glow your skin has naturally at this age.

You've got it—so show it off!

The same advice holds true for treatment products. Unless you have an especially sensitive skin condition, you don't need many. And you don't need your mother's! Don't get into her cosmetics bag—not for makeup, and not for treatment products. If you start using a cream formulated for forty-year-old skin now, what are you going to use later? I'm not saying you should ignore treatment products. Even if your complexion is perfection, you should always cleanse, tone, and moisturize. Well-treated skin always ages more gracefully. However, you should seek out products that protect your skin rather than recondition it. Be wary of overcorrecting oiliness with astringents that are too drying. And use only a light, water-based moisturizer.

Your daytime makeup routine can be as simple as moisturize/blot/powder. Add color with eye pencils, mascara, and blusher. At this age, you can use a lot of different colors around the eyes. Work with pencils, and blend with your fingertips. Choose mascara in a coordinating color. There's time enough for blacks and browns later in life!

Follow your natural blush when you apply cheek color. It looks younger when it's high and right on the cheek pillows. You might brush it lightly across the bridge of your nose, too, for a sunstruck look. Avoid any detailed sculpting of your face at this stage. Your makeup will look too premeditated.

Keep your lips natural-looking. One of my favorite tricks is to scratch a little powder blusher with a fingertip and apply it right to the lips. Then lightly gloss. Too many young women pile the gloss on for a "natural look,"

Renee Simonsen's flawless complexion needs virtually no coverage for a naturally radiant daytime look—just a hint of earthy-colored blush to give her cheeks a healthy glow.

Incredibly big, blue eyes are the focus of Kim Alexis's nighttime look, and accentuating her prominent cheekbones with bright blush gives a more dramatic look.

but this is the farthest thing from it! Gloss is best when you use just a touch, then lightly blot most of it away.

Even if your best beauty look is natural by day, you can—and should—add a little sophistication in the evening. This doesn't mean covering your face with a heavy matte makeup. You still want your skin's natural radiance to show through. Use a translucent powder or blusher to heighten the glow, then concentrate on the eyes. Make them more dramatic by using eye shadow colors in addition to pencils all around your eyes. Bring out your blusher a bit more, adding a touch of color at the temples and chin for a more glowing look.

And, please, no unfinished lips! Even if you never wear lipstick at all by day, you have to give your lips some attention to balance the extra eye makeup. You can keep your lip color pale, if that's what you like, but your lips must look finished. When they do, it's always true that the eyes become even more important. Just try it and see. It works like magic!

A TIME FOR EXPERIMENTATION: 25–35

As you move into your late twenties, it's time to pull out all the stops. You are physically at your most beautiful; your skin is firm; the wrinkles and shadows have yet to set in. You are at an age where your makeup can be a bit more dramatic without making you look too old. It can be a bit more experimental without making you look too young. You should try everything—any new color, any new technique that catches your interest. Your face, your makeup, your colors should not be "set." You're never going to have a better canvas to create on, and somewhere in your experimentation you're going to find a few faces that will make you look better than you've ever seen yourself.

It's also important at this stage to monitor your treatment regimen carefully. You've got to do all you can to guard against the wrinkles that will come. You can't prevent them, but if you continue to treat your skin with care, you may postpone them. You should upgrade your skin care regimen from purely protective products to include treatment ones as well. Begin using beauty masks keyed to your skin type once a month. Make sure your makeup formulations aren't too drying. If your skin isn't staying soft and supple year round, start your search *now* for products that will keep it that way.

Guard against any unnecessary damage to the skin. Overexposure to the sun can really speed up the aging process, and that's the last thing you need. Select a base with a sunscreen for light protection (most only have a

Because Isabella Rossellini's face is so full of character, all she needs for a sophisticated but simple daytime look is a bit of definition around the eyes and a strong mouth.

Iman's inborn elegance and
sophistication enable her to wear lots
of makeup at night without looking
overdone; iridescent shadows and
deep, strong colors just enhance her
dramatic look.

sun protection factor of 4); and a serious sun-screen (above 15) any time your face will be directly exposed. Apply it right under your makeup to block the ultraviolet rays that damage collagen, the substance that keeps the skin firm and smooth. Changes that are interpreted as signs of aging are often only the visible evidence of sun damage.

If you simply must have that tanned, "healthy" glow, a bronzer or a translucent gel applied over a sunscreen will give you the same effect—without the consequences.

A seasonless makeup for you includes moisturizer, base, and powder. You can be more vibrant in the touches of color on your cheeks and lips. For your eyes, you can work with any kind of shadows you like, but don't harden your face with too much color. Always remember that less is more. At this stage, corrective shading will not look too artificial, as long as everything is well blended.

Be as exciting as you can be in the evening. Now is the time to do the most dramatic makeup of your life. Play with colors, highlights, shadows. Sweep highlighting blush in a C-curve from your cheekbone to your brow-bone. Use dark, dramatic colors around the eyes—and lots of mascara. Make your blush and your lipstick bright. This is your time to be absolutely dazzling!

BEAUTY CONSOLIDATION: 35–50

You know who you are by now; your likes and dislikes reflect themselves in the clothes you choose to wear, in the way you choose to look. Your beauty image is more than physical. It is an amalgam of your looks plus your personality. One has stamped itself upon the other, and the two cannot be separated.

You bring your inner resources, your own natural beauty, and your life experiences to this consolidation. And the result is a much more interesting, womanly appearance. You no longer have the physical perfection you had at twenty-five, but something far richer is evident in your face. You'll destroy it if you try to look younger. Nobody wants you to. Don't claim as your own every new color, every trendy trick. Don't take your makeup cues from rock videos, or from your daughter. If the impulse to wear yellow lipstick and blue nails hits you, resist it—even at Halloween!

You'd do better to spend your money on a facial. Now is the time to give your skin regular treats. Go for a professional peeling mask to rid the skin of dulling, dead surface cells. Switch from a one-night-only beauty mask to a longer-lasting treatment mask. And don't be discouraged if you don't see results right away. It took a long while to happen. Your skin's not going to rejuvenate overnight.

The best things you can do for your beauty come from within. Bring back the glow by improving your circulation; get enough cardiovascular exercise; use a stimulating shower or tub jet; slough your skin with a body loofah;

Lee Remick has a classic elegance that calls for subtlety in the makeup she chooses for day: light base, subdued colors that are saved from looking somber by a bright shade of lipstick.

The planes of Diahann Carroll's face
are wonderful to highlight for a
sophisticated evening makeup, and lots
of lashes make her expressive eyes
look even bigger.

have a massage to tingle from head to toe. Be good to yourself, and you'll look the better for it. Don't forget proper diet and rest. Mistreatment will show faster on your skin than it ever has before.

Pay more attention to special-interest areas of your body. One all-purpose cream may not be enough to restore, soften, and firm *everything*. You'll need a richer, thicker cream for your neck and décolletage; a lighter cream for the delicate undereye area; and a night cream that's heavy enough to hold in your skin's moisture.

By day you should look cared for, soignée. Always use moisturizer, base, and powder. Lift off any excess powder that gets trapped under the eyes with the pillow tip of your little finger. Gently rim the eye area with it after you have powdered. Bring back a little natural glow by pressing a cotton ball, lightly dampened with astringent, to your makeup (avoid the nose area).

Use more natural-colored eye shadows on your lids. Browns, taupes, prunes, and peaches are softer. If you want to use a definite color, keep it subdued. Blue is fine if it's a navy blue, not a bright cobalt blue. Add brightness with your cheek and lip colors.

There are ways to brighten your look for evening without resorting to obviously bright colors. Strategically placed highlighter, for instance, will bring out your eyes better than brighter eye shadow shades. Place a dot of highlight shadow just under the arch of the brow and at the center of the lid. Don't streak it across the entire lid—and don't use iridescent shadows. Make your eyes more dramatic with lots of mascara, but be sure to comb lashes well between layers. A too-thick mascara will make you look hard.

Sculpt any unwanted change in your facial shape with color, blending well. In the evening, keep your accent colors vibrant but not shocking. Let the woman you've become shine through.

CONTINUING BEAUTY: 50+

Don't try to change your image as you get older; it won't suit the personality that's developed along with it. If you were a classic beauty when you were younger, you will still be a classic beauty, no matter what your age. If you were a sophisticated, vibrant beauty, you will always be sophisticated, though perhaps a little less vibrant in the colors you choose to play up your style. If you were a natural, outdoorsy woman, you're not going to suddenly turn into a painted lady.

The one thing you must do, however, is to accommodate your makeup routine to the changes that are taking place. If you ignore them, you'll date yourself forever. The structure and the texture of your face will soften with age; your makeup must soften too.

Even more important than the makeup you select is the treatment regimen you follow. Once again, your skin becomes your most important asset. You need more than mere moisturizing creams. You need creams that are formulated to rejuvenate skin and renew cells. And don't forget skin-freshening masks. Although your skin may be thinner and more fragile now, the gentler freshening masks will treat it kindly.

For evening, Joan Fontaine's graceful, sophisticated makeup is applied with a light hand. Her eyes are not made up, but rather they are designed with delicate pencil strokes.

My mother, Helene Jacobs, is proof that scrupulous attention to skin really pays off. Now all she needs for a casual but elegant daytime look is a bit of mascara, a touch of eyebrow pencil, and a flattering shade of lipstick.

Look for thicker, oilier night creams. Your skin needs that kind of nourishment. Creams that are 80 percent water will evaporate and won't do you a bit of good. But don't put a thick cream on right before you get into bed, or it will "plump up" during the night. Put it on a good half-hour before bedtime, then watch the news, brush your teeth, write a note—anything to fill the time so you won't be tempted to lie down with an oily face. After your half-hour wait, blot off any excess.

You may think you've reached the age where you needn't worry so much about makeup. That's only partially true. You can wear less if you choose, but any makeup you do wear should be perfectly applied. A careless job will only emphasize everything you want to hide. Errors will immediately become obvious: lipstick that doesn't follow the mouth; blush that's in the wrong place; powder that's too heavy.

If you wish to rely on the beauty of your skin and avoid makeup altogether, I suggest you still use a moisturizer and—always—a powder. Even a transparent powder is better than none. Contrary to popular myth, shine does not make you look more youthful. The highlights that shine casts only accentuate the shadows caused by wrinkles.

For more hints on creating the most youthful makeup, see the "Tips to Look 10 Years Better" section in this chapter. The general rule to remember is: softly natural by day; stronger but still subtle by night.

The best makeup for day consists of a moisturizer, base, powder, blusher, mascara, and lipstick. Use products that are light to the touch. They can be sheer, fluid, or transparent.

For blusher, a cream formulation is less drying than a powder. Place it high, in the center of your cheek pillows. Save the powder blusher for dotting just a small amount of color on your eyelids—it livens up the skin tone and makes your eyes sparkle. Avoid other eye shadow colors in this area, especially anything iridescent. Go to a softer shade of mascara—gray or brown is better than black. A light layer of mascara just on the top lashes will look far more youthful than any elaborate shadowing technique. If your eyebrows are too dark for your face—or hair—have them lightened professionally. Nothing is more disconcerting than two dark lines across a soft face. If the color of your brows is fine as is, don't draw them in too heavily. Lighter is younger.

Keep your lips soft and pink. If necessary, outline them subtly, with pencil to keep the color from "bleeding" into the tiny lines around the mouth. Do not modify the shape of the lips in any way. Use two coats of a luminous, natural-looking lipstick, blotting each coat with a makeup tissue. A softer shade is younger than a brighter one.

The colors you choose—from base to blusher to lipstick—should all have a pink undertone. Anything with yellow in it is aging, and unflattering. Avoid orange, brown, and red lipsticks and anything green for the eyes.

Always be light-handed in your application. Any excess in makeup always makes a woman look older. Be particularly careful with powder. If it is too heavily applied, it will collect in all the wrong places. If it is too pale, it will put an unattractive accent on the teeth (especially if they are not white-white).

Evening makeup should brighten your entire face without making you appear vampish or overly dramatic. An overdone face calls attention to the makeup, rather than to how attractive you look. You can achieve just the right intensity by brightening your blusher and your lip color by one or two shades. Add excitement to your eyes with a dot of highlight shadow in the center of the lid, just above the lashline. Too much color on the eyes will create too harsh a contrast with softer skin or lighter hair. Again, avoid iridescent shadow like the plague, and keep your mascara layers light. Thickening your lashes will only create a dark veil around your eyes.

Don't forget dowager's tricks! Pearls around the neck or ruby-and-diamond chokers aren't for ostentation only. A light, bright color, a white scarf, something expensive and sparkling—all can work wonders to brighten your entire face!

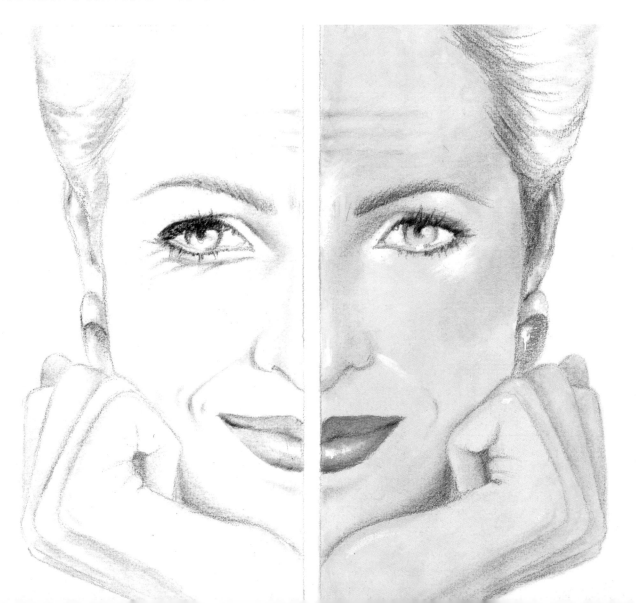

Tips to Look 10 Years Better

No matter what your chronological age, your face may feel slightly ahead of its time. If that's the case, there are certain things to watch for.

Base

The ideal color for a rested and fresh-looking complexion is a pinky beige. Select a base in a shade slightly lighter than your natural skin tone. A fluid base is better than a thick, covering makeup that molds to your face and accentuates all the imperfections of your skin.

Concealer

Choose a cover-up that is close to the color of your base. The two should blend perfectly. White circles around your eyes will only make you look sad. You can also use concealer to smooth eyelids before you apply makeup and keep them fresher-looking.

Blusher

Use a luminous, creamy blusher instead of a dry-looking powder blusher. Add color high on the cheek pillows. Do not sculpt hollows.

Eye Shadow

Avoid all creamy eye shadows. They will melt and accumulate in the folds of the eyelid. Use soft, subtle colors around your eyes. Avoid obvious black and all iridescents.

Eye Liner

Use only a brown or gray pencil and blend with a cotton swab. A liquid liner gives too harsh a line and is too difficult to apply. A kohl pencil will give your eyes a heavy expression. Never go inside the rim of the lid when you are lining.

Eyebrows

Lighten brows one or two tones if your hair has gone light (for whatever reason). But don't go overboard. If your eyebrows are too light, it will take away your expression. If they're too thin, your makeup will look dated. To accent, use only a taupe or a chestnut pencil (never brown or black).

Lip Color

Choose lipstick with a luminous color and a transparent texture. Pay attention to the formulation: Lipsticks with softening or protective ingredients will help prevent drying and chapping. Soft, smooth lips always look younger. After forty, you should outline lips with a pencil to keep color from "bleeding" into tiny cracks, keeping the color of your outline pencil as close to your lipstick shade as possible. Never make the outline obvious or modify the natural shape of the lips.

Powder

Choose powder with a transparent quality. It will obtain the exact color of your base without darkening it. If you prefer a tinted powder, do not use one that's paler than your base. Always powder gently. To avoid accentuating wrinkles, press powder only on the middle of your face; dust it *lightly* over the mobile zones.

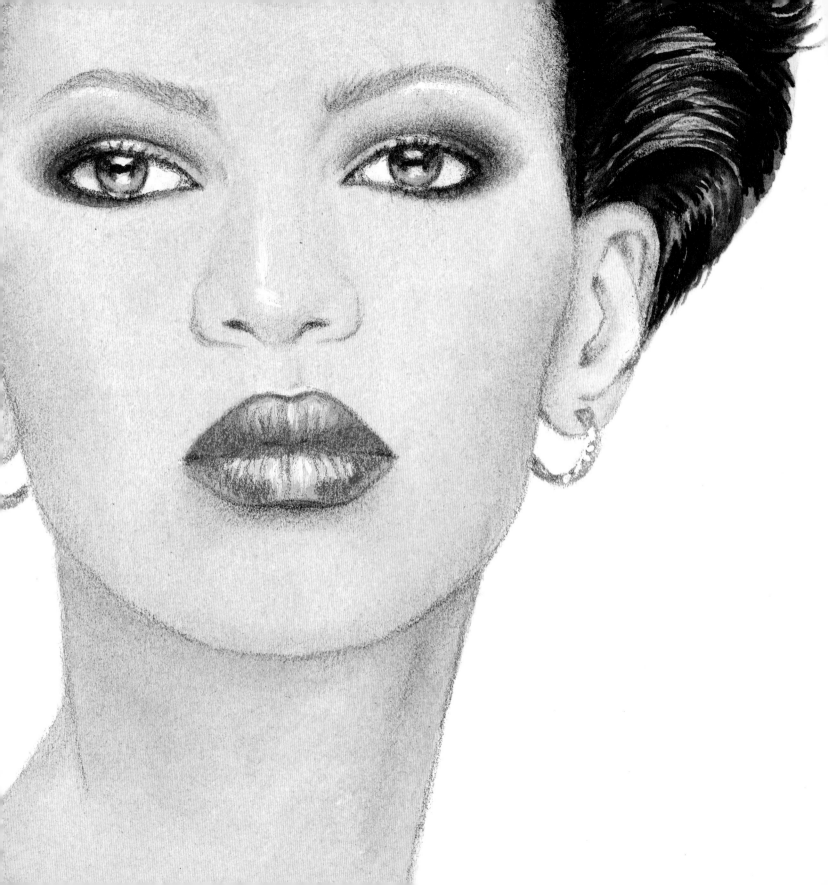

Makeup for Black Women

Naturally, skin pigmentation plays a large part in determining the shades you select for your face. But that's not the whole story. The evenness of skin color and the structure of facial features must also be taken into consideration. Special attention must be paid to unifying skin tone, downplaying overly prominent features, and focusing on the upper third of the face. In general, there are three areas black women should emphasize and three areas to watch out for.

Eyes

Accent your eyes, but avoid light, powdery colors. They look like flour on darker skin. Work, instead, with dark browns, prunes, and burgundies. Use a small dot of iridescent highlighter just under the arch of the brow and at the center of the lid. Never stroke iridescent color over the entire eyelid. To give your eyes some evening glamour, lightly brush colorless, loose translucent powder over the lid. The subtle glow in the powder should be enough.

Nose

If you have a wide nose, you don't want it to be the focal point of your face. To slim it, shade the nose at the sides with a darker base. Look for other correcting techniques in Chapter 4. And avoid attention-getting shine! Always, always powder.

Cheeks

The touch of color you add to your cheeks is very important. It will give a focus to your whole face. Stay away from orange tones; they don't look natural or healthy. Instead, choose reds, pinks, or burgundies. The same holds true for lip and nail colors. Review the face-shaping techniques described in Chapter 4 to find out how to place cheek color to your best advantage.

Complexion

Black skin rarely has a unified tone, and it is often without brightness. A base will battle both conditions. Select one a shade lighter than your normal skin tone, plus another base a tone darker for shading. Black skin tends to reject makeup, so make the effect last longer by avoiding oil-based products. They'll slide right off your skin. And always use a powder, one that is either transparent (to take on the color of the base) or slightly tinted to correct a yellow or gray undertone (page 30).

Brows

Emphasize your brows, but never use a black pencil alone—no matter what their natural color. Use gray or a mixture of gray and black pencils.

Lips

Always apply base first to even the color. Then powder before you apply lipstick. See Chapter 4 for techniques to correct any problems in shape.

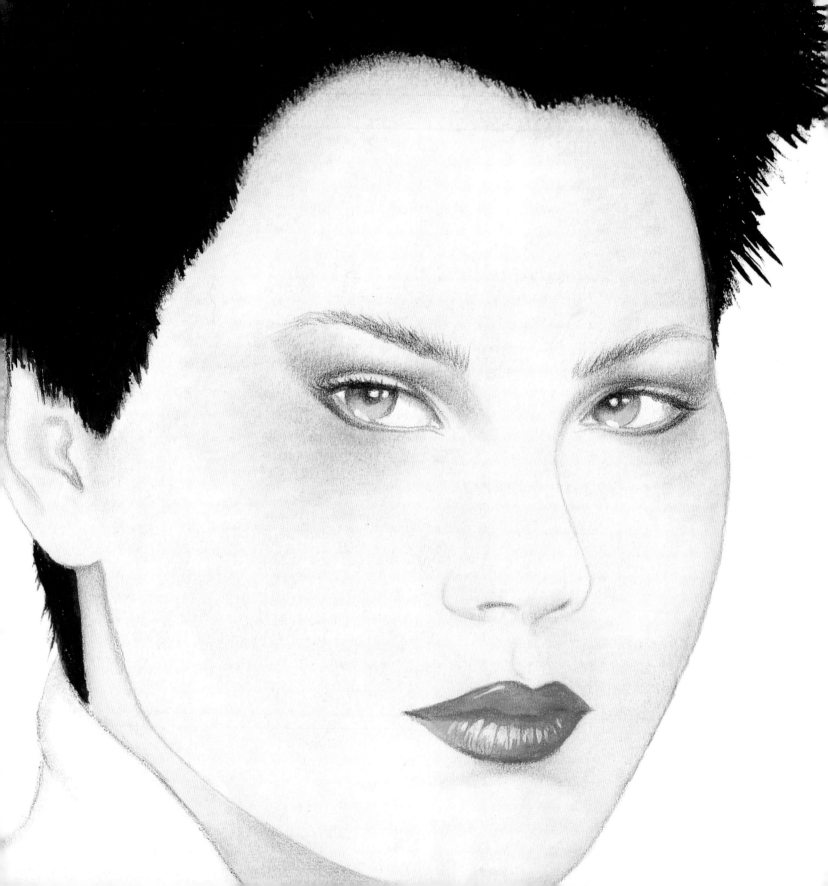

Makeup for Asian Women

Asian skin tone can be enhanced if the right colors are chosen to complement it. The trick is first to neutralize any tendency to sallowness with a beige base. Then go to the warm side of the palette for touches of color. Choose earth tones, corals, bright reds, or natural browns. Do *not* think pink; it's not the best shade for Asian skin.

Eyes

Stay with blacks, browns, and earthy colors for shadow shades. Add yellow or gold only as a highlighter.

Bring out the bridge of your nose by using a dark brown color (use eye shadow, powder, or cream, but nothing iridescent), applying it from the inner corner of your eye to just under the brow. Blend toward the outside corner of the eye. Rim the entire eye with a black pencil and smudge.

Shape the lower part of the eye by drawing a straight line below the lashes, starting a quarter of the way away from the inner corner. Take it straight across, and angle it up at the end. From the inner corner of the eye to the point where this line begins, curve a small line upward. Then follow the instructions for makeup for a narrow eyelid in Chapter 4.

Cheeks

Emphasize the cheekbones by placing your color very high, right on top of the cheek pillows.

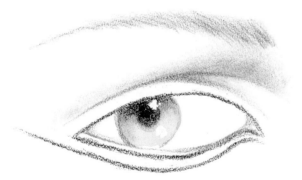
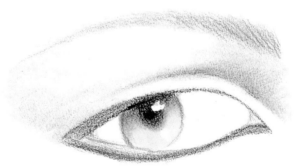

Makeup for Women with White Hair

White hair is a color; it is not an age. But too many people think one condition automatically indicates the other. Nonsense. I've seen as many youthful women with white hair as I've seen older women with blond hair. Or red. Or brown. Or black. In this age of hair-coloring technology, a woman doesn't *have* to have white hair—unless it is flattering to her. And it can be very flattering, at any age! But it does call for special makeup techniques.

To begin with, white hair provides no frame for the face. Hair of any other color creates a frame, one that softens or hardens your features. White hair is too neutral to either soften or harden your face. That means, for better or for worse, your face takes the spotlight. It becomes the focal point. And you must be very careful what you do with it. Any makeup that is too aggressive or too blatant will be even more jarring than it would be on a woman whose hair color can counteract the effect. Here are some techniques that will work well for you.

Eyes
Lots of mascara, rather than a lot of colorful eye shadow, will give eyes the best emphasis. Work closer to the eye, rather than extending the color to surround the eye.

Lips
Your mouth is your strongest focal point. It's centralized, and it doesn't compete with the absence of color in your hair. Choose clear, bright shades, but not shocking ones.

Base
Keep the face pale, toward the pink side. Stay away from yellows.

Cheeks
Keep the color focused toward the center of the face rather than extending it to the hairline. The contrast between bright blusher and white hair is too severe.

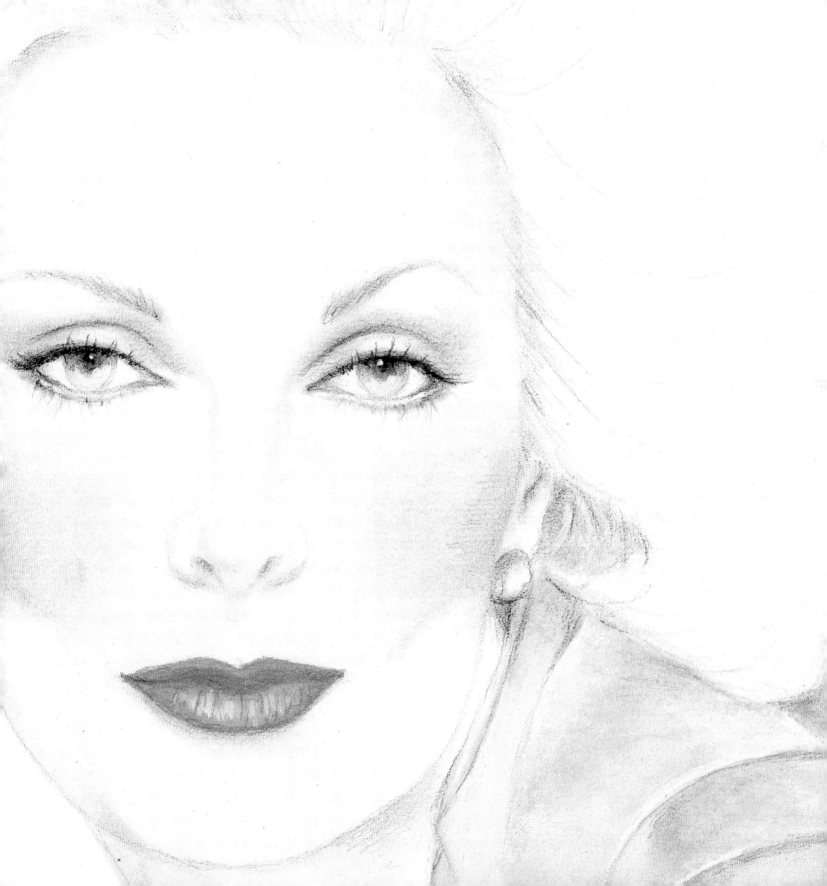

Makeup for Women Who Wear Eyeglasses

No matter how lightweight, clear, or visually nonexistent eyeglass frames are, they are going to throw a slight shadow on your face. So you must pay particular attention to your eye makeup. And this is the one time I'm going to suggest some exaggeration—just a bit. You need to bring your eyes out just a little more than most women. If you don't wear eye makeup as a rule, do so when you wear your glasses. Or intensify the colors and strengthen the application of the makeup you normally wear. But this doesn't give you permission to go overboard. Anything too dark, too dramatic, is going to draw the wrong kind of attention to your eyes. Be especially careful if you wear magnifying (far-sighted) corrective lenses.

The secret is to *lighten* the entire eye area. Begin by brushing on a light concealer color in the shape of your glasses, going from just under the brows to the lower rim of the eye socket. Then powder. Apply your base and the rest of your makeup in the normal manner.

Oval

As with makeup, an oval face can get away with anything—rectangular, square, round, or triangular frames; thick frames, thin frames, wide frames, or narrow ones.

Square

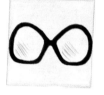

To soften the angles of the face, look for gently curved frames. You don't want anything wide, rectangular, or overextended. The lenses can reach below the cheekbones.

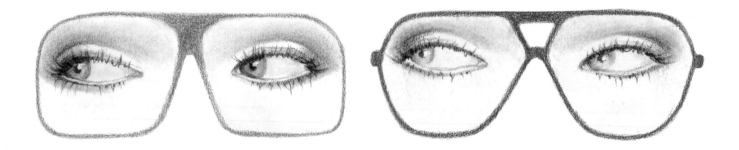

When it comes time to do your eyes, underline and shadow in the best way for their shape, as discussed in Chapter 4. Just remember to keep the colors you select in the lighter range.

Reverse your play-it-up technique when you reach for the mascara. If applied too heavily, it will make dirty smudges behind the lenses. Mascaras with fibers can be messy too.

When it comes to your eyebrows, two are enough! Never let them show above your eyeglass frames, or you'll look like you have four. Your eyebrows should either be hidden by the frames or follow their shape.

The frames you select and their color can enhance—or hide—a multitude of facial features. And their shape undeniably influences the proportion of your face.

Eyeglass frames can perform other tricks too. A low bridge will shorten a long nose; a high bridge will elongate a short nose. You can narrow the space between your eyes with a darker-colored bridge. And if your eyes are too close together, you'll want a colorless bridge. The very color of your frames can be a great complexion booster. Choose pink or salmon to brighten a sallow complexion; gray, pale green, or blue to soften a rosy one. The general color rule to remember is: *Lighter frames for lighter hair.*

Round

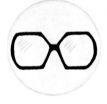

Look for angular aviators or geometrically shaped frames. Anything too wide will echo the roundness of your face.

Long

A frame that divides the face horizontally is your best bet. Big, face-hiding frames are fine, as long as they are deep from top to bottom, not wide from side to side. A frame that extends beyond the sides of your face will make the narrowness more apparent.

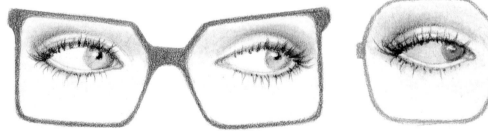

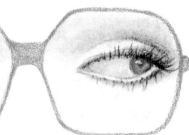

Fantasy Makeup

You may want a colorful face for an evening makeup. But for the biggest evenings, take it one step farther—into the realm of pure fantasy. A fantasy face is for those times when you want an extraordinary, imaginative, all-eyes-on-you look. It might be for an extravagant occasion, like a masquerade ball, a New Year's party, or a Mardi Gras carnival. Or it might be just to add an intriguing touch to last year's basic black dress. Whatever the reason, it's your time to shine.

To create a fantasy face, you need to work with new colors—and work in new ways. Don't think in terms of eye shadow, lipstick, blusher. Think only of *color*. Look at every item in your makeup drawer as potential "paint" for any area of your face. As mentioned earlier, you become an artist the moment you begin to apply *any* makeup. Well, this time you're going to become an artist extraordinaire!

You've got to look at your face as well as your makeup in a whole new way. Don't see an eye, a nose, a mouth. Look only for angles, curves, planes. You're going to put makeup where it's never gone before. And you can use the basic architecture of your face to determine the perfect placement for your design. Don't go against your bone structure. Plan your design to accent the natural contours. Looking at Cubist paintings or Picasso's women might inspire you.

First, figure out what you are going to do with your hair for the evening. An upswept style works best with upward makeup strokes.

Hair that falls closely around the face puts the nix on intricate cheek designs. If you're painting your face, you must always think of the frame.

Next, pick the colors you need for the effect you want to create. Naturally, what you are wearing may influence your final selection of shades. But this time forget about coordinating color with your skin tone, eye color, and hair color. You don't want your strokes of fantasy to blend into any natural harmony-of-color scheme. The point is to let the color stand out. Going for a shocker? Try a hot fuchsia/bright yellow/royal blue combination. Want to create a softer effect? Team up turquoise/lime green/deep purple. Something for a bang-up Fourth of July celebration? Nothing's better than red/white/blue. For maximum glamour, go for the golds, or mix gold with black and silver. And don't forget the glitter!

Try your color choices out side by side on a piece of paper—before you streak them across your face—to make sure they're going to give you the impact you want. You should also practice drawing your design a few times. And remember, anything goes. Be as original as you want. A simple, single motif is the most effective. You might just add swipes of bright color in unexpected spots: a dash of blue from your eyebrow to your forehead, a swirl of yellow just at the top of your cheek. Never try to do too much in too many places.

For a whimsical touch, you might pick up a design idea from the dress you are wearing.

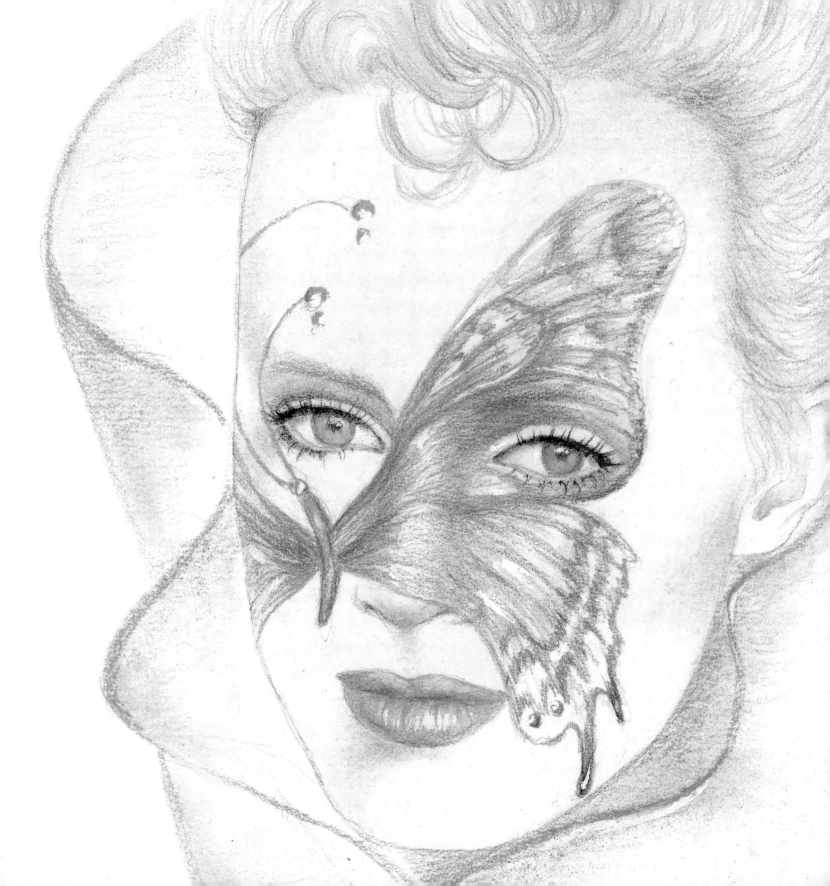

Whatever you do, the final result should embellish you—not make you ugly. Here are some ideas to try:

Lightning flash
Fireworks
Waterfall
Vines and leaves
Stripes
Stars
Clouds
Swirls
Zebra stripes
Fish
Checkerboard
Butterflies
Teardrops
Triangles
Geometric shapes
Spider web
Gilded eye patch

Once you have confidence in your design and have selected your colors you can begin on your skin. Here are the steps to creating the face of your wildest fantasies.

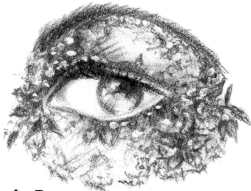

1. Apply Base
Have your makeup completed through the base stage. After all, the parts of your face that aren't being "designed" should look perfectly normal. And once you begin creating your fantasy look, it will be impossible to slip the base under it or around it.

2. Draw Your Design
Draw everything in with a light makeup pencil. Use a pale gray, light brown, or soft pink.

Once you are certain you have the placement exactly the way you want it, go over the outline with the color pencils of your choice.

3. Powder Over
After the basic design is drawn, dust on powder. Use a soft, thick brush. (A rolling, press/release motion would be the end of everything!)

4. Color In
Fill in your design outline with color. It's best to use a thin brush and makeup with a creamy consistency. Cream eye shadow, cream blush, and cream lip colors make it easier to paint on just the right amount—and the right intensity—of color. Also, if you choose to add glitter as a final touch, cream formulations will hold better.

5. Start Sparkling!
Glitter adds exciting sparkle to a fantasy face, especially if you use it to emphasize the edges of your design. But you must apply it carefully, well away from your eyes. Don't use any sort of glue on your skin to make it stick. And don't —ever—just throw it on. Have patience! Dampen a tiny brush, touch it to the glitter, then apply it directly on top of your creamy color. It should last long enough to get you through the evening.

You can't "fix" a fantasy makeup with powder, or the whole effect will be lost in the mist. The best trick for ensuring its longevity is to apply thin, even layers that won't flake or crack. Keep in mind that you're an artist, not a graffiti painter!

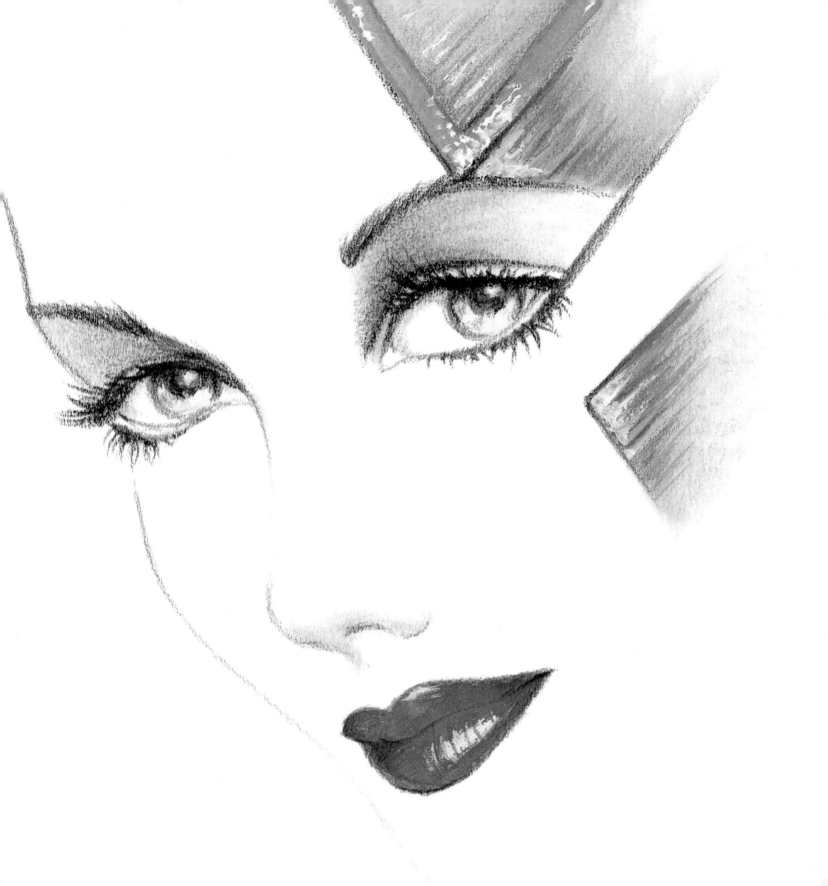

Planet Faces

Certain characteristics—physical as well as emotional—can sometimes be very recognizable across a whole segment of people. It's easy to say there are "types," but why *do* some people share so many similarities? Is it heredity? Nationality? Date of birth? Believers in the power of astral signs have long attributed their traits to the influence of the stars. But just as beauty and temperament often go hand in hand, it is just as easy to identify a planetary influence on personality, behavior, and physical characteristics.

Want to explore a whole new way of analyzing your beauty and your behavior? Find out what kind of "planet face" is most like yours!

MARS

<u>FACE</u> Often square, strong

<u>MOUTH</u> Tends to be thin

<u>NOSE</u> Prominent, sometimes with a high arch

<u>EYES</u> Green, often deep set

<u>EYEBROWS</u> Thick

<u>HAIR</u> Red, bronze

<u>COMPLEXION</u> Ruddy

<u>HEIGHT</u> Tall

<u>ATTITUDE</u> Provocative

<u>PERSONALITY TRAITS</u> Often impatient, quick-tempered, mercurial; equally open and devoted

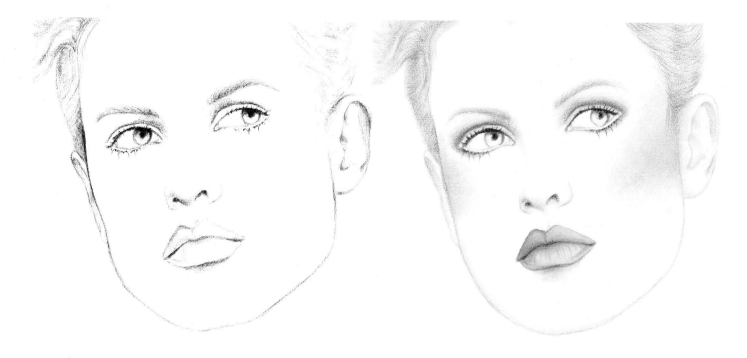

Mars, god of war, is dominating you, and the influence is noticeable in both your personality and your physical appearance. You are likely to have an angular face, a slender silhouette, long legs, and slim hips. You have strong, straight teeth, which you often reveal—in anger and in friendship. You love sports, especially highly competitive, physically exhausting ones. You are not afraid of rougher contact sports and would never worry about breaking a nail. No one can advise you to be strong and firm; you already are. But you must also learn the discreet charm of adding softness and gentleness to your appearance.

Best Makeup

Do everything you can to soften your face and coloring. Start with a beige base and curve the angles of your face with blush. Put color very high on the cheekbones, and on the chin. Soften the jawline with a curve of darker correcting color. You must bring your eyes out to create a new focus for your face. Begin by tweezing unruly brows, but make sure that you don't shorten their length. Remove hairs only to create a harmonious arch. Then lighten the entire eye area with concealer. Use a touch of pale eye color on your lids, then rim the eyes with a dark pencil. Add a dark shadow in the crease of the lid. Draw your mouth big and laughing!

119

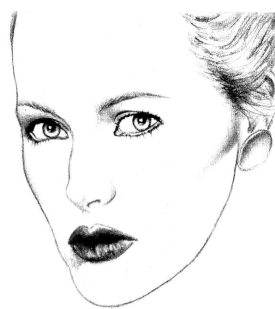

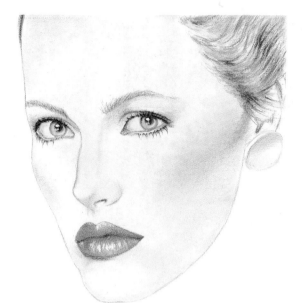

SATURN

<u>FACE</u> Long, often narrow

<u>MOUTH</u> Can turn down at the corners

<u>NOSE</u> Thin, sometimes with a low hook

<u>EYES</u> Dark, often with droopy lids

<u>EYEBROWS</u> Arched, with a downward line at the end

<u>HAIR</u> Dark

<u>COMPLEXION</u> Pale, slightly sallow

<u>HEIGHT</u> Tall

<u>ATTITUDE</u> Composed

<u>PERSONALITY TRAITS</u> Intelligent, distrustful, wistful; tenacious and faithful

It is easy to misinterpret the downward angles of your face. Although some may view you as doleful and pessimistic, you are actually revealing strength of concentration and determination. Discretion is important to you: in your clothes, your movements, your actions. Your taste and style tend toward the classic. You would rather be considered serious than frivolous—but it's time you took a little light-hearted beauty advice!

Best Makeup
Use your concentration to brighten your appearance. You must open up your face and give it some splendor. Bring your complexion to life with a light, luminous base. Give your cheeks more attention by creating width with a brighter blush. Place it right on the cheekbone, and blend upward toward the temples. Lift the ends of your eyebrows by tweezing and redesigning the line. Use a light accent shadow under the browbone, covering the entire lid area. Iridescent shadows are the ones for you. Remember, you want to add a little glow anywhere you can. Choose a luminous lipstick, and tilt the color up at the corners.

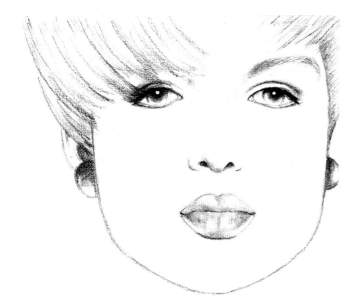

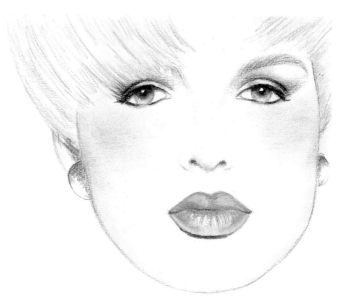

MOON

<u>FACE</u> Round

<u>MOUTH</u> Small and round, tilted up at the corners

<u>NOSE</u> Upturned

<u>EYES</u> Pale

<u>EYEBROWS</u> Rounded and high

<u>HAIR</u> Light to ashen brown

<u>COMPLEXION</u> Noticeably pale

<u>HEIGHT</u> Petite to average

<u>ATTITUDE</u> Agitated

<u>PERSONALITY TRAITS</u> Versatile, changeable, sometimes quixotic; imaginative, given to flights of fantasy

The moon does play tricks on you. You can go from moody to mercurial in seconds. But you are usually forgiven, because when the air clears you are often smiling, giggling, laughing. Your face, which can be quite pretty, is always very feminine. And you can be quite sensual. At times, your dreamy quality makes you seem ethereal, otherworldly. To bring yourself back down to earth, add some reality to your beauty look.

Best Makeup
Balance the roundness of your face with a slightly tanned base. Use a darker correcting color at the temples and jawline. Don't bring your blush too far out; keep it centered. Lower your brows by bringing eye shadow up higher on your lid, all the way to the browline. Try to make your brows appear thicker and more horizontal. Tweeze them at the ends so they do not curve down. Rim your eyes with a darker color just at the lashline. Let your hair fall naturally. A contrived style does not suit your personality.

SUN

<u>FACE</u> Oval or full

<u>MOUTH</u> Well designed

<u>NOSE</u> Straight and slightly arched

<u>EYES</u> Light

<u>EYEBROWS</u> Lightly arched, well placed

<u>HAIR</u> Light

<u>COMPLEXION</u> In the pink range

<u>HEIGHT</u> Average

<u>ATTITUDE</u> Elegant

<u>PERSONALITY TRAITS</u> Emotional, impractical, impetuous; creative and authoritative

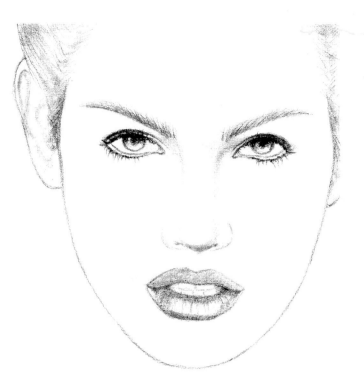

You don't pass unnoticed. The way you look, the way you move, draws attention from everyone else in the room. Your movements are slow and deliberate, yet graceful. Your gestures are ample, expansive. The language of your body reveals both a liking for power and the ability to command it. You are most content when you are in total control of any situation. Your physical attributes reflect your strength. Your body is firm, not skinny. Your shoulders are strong. Your hair is radiant and healthy. Since you are usually at the peak of your form, the only beauty advice for you is to have more fun, more fantasy.

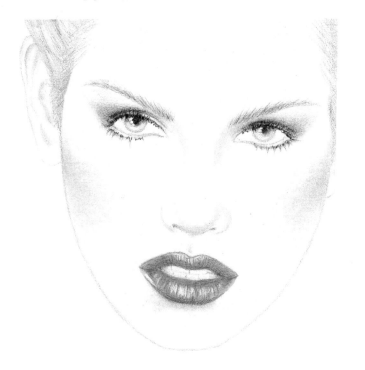

Best Makeup

Stay with the natural look you love. Avoid a thick base; the effect is too sophisticated for you. Narrow the fullness of your face with a darker base along the jawline. Then blush from the cheekbones to the temple, at the sides of the forehead, and on the chin. Don't be afraid to add eye color. It won't look as artificial as you think. Just avoid the obvious. Your best shades are warm nuances of color: taupes, browns, cinnamons, rusts, burgundies, golds, beiges. Brush your eyebrows straight up to soften your face. And let your hair fly!

Acknowledgments

Our gratitude to Carol Southern and Pam Krauss, our beautifully insightful editors, and to the following wonderful women who permitted Rex to illustrate their beauty:

Anouk Aimée
Kim Alexis
Amalia
Ariane
Carmen
Diahann Carroll
Joan Fontaine
Iman
Lee Remick
Isabella Rossellini
Brooke Shields
Renee Simonsen